Multiple Sclerosis - Pathways, Diagnosis and Therapeutic Targets

Edited by Liam Chen

Published in London, United Kingdom

Multiple Sclerosis - Pathways, Diagnosis and Therapeutic Targets
http://dx.doi.org/10.5772/intechopen.1005720
Edited by Liam Chen

Contributors
Alexander Kolsanov, Alexander Zakharov, Bhupendra O. Khatri, Danyelly Bruneska Gondim Martins, Elena Khivintseva, Eleni Litsou, Esra Demir Unal, Henrik Hasseldam, Igor Shirolapov, Irina Andreevna Vyshlova, Jay S. Raval, Jordana Marina da Silva, Kleiton de Barros Borges, Maria Helena Menezes Estevam Alves, Mariya Sergeeva, Natalia Romanchuk, Olga Pavlova, Sergey Mikhailovich Karpov, Valéria Visani, Victória Regina da Silva, Xinchen Nie, Yawei Liu, Yulia Komarova

First published in London, United Kingdom, 2025 by IntechOpen
IntechOpen is the global imprint of INTECHOPEN LIMITED, registered in England and Wales, registration number: 11086078, 167-169 Great Portland Street, London, W1W 5PF, United Kingdom

For EU product safety concerns: IN TECH d.o.o., Prolaz Marije Krucifikse Kozulić 3, 51000 Rijeka, Croatia, info@intechopen.com or visit our website at intechopen.com.

British Library Cataloguing-in-Publication Data
A catalogue record for this book is available from the British Library

Multiple Sclerosis - Pathways, Diagnosis and Therapeutic Targets
Edited by Liam Chen
p. cm.

This title is part of the Nervous System and Mental Health Book Series, Volume 1
Series Editor: Toshikazu Shinba

Print ISBN 978-1-83634-710-1
Online ISBN 978-1-83634-709-5
eBook (PDF) ISBN 978-1-83634-711-8
ISSN 3050-2985

If disposing of this product, please recycle the paper responsibly.

IntechOpen Book Series

Nervous System and Mental Health

Volume 1

Aims and Scope of the Series

Mental health is frequently linked to the nervous system. Conversely, disturbances in the nervous system often lead to mental health problems. However, this linkage is not as clear as it is commonly accepted. Mental health is usually described using subjective terms, which are based on psychological and psychiatric symptomatology. Diagnosis of a mental illness is made through the presence of the subjective symptoms characterizing the illness.

On the other hand, the nervous system has been deeply investigated using objective measures, including molecular, genetic, imaging, pharmacological and physiological ones. It is essential to combine objective views of the nervous system with subjective perspectives on mental health to develop an integrative approach to understanding human cognitive functions and achieving overall well-being. In this book series, experts in various fields of the nervous system and mental health will present their views on these challenging topics.

Meet the Series Editor

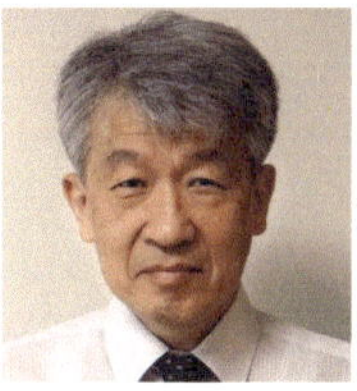

Dr. Toshikazu Shinba is a psychiatrist and neuroscientist who has been working in both clinical and basic research fields. He has been affiliated with the Tokyo Institute of Psychiatry, Department of Neurophysiology and Stress Disorders Project, and now works as a psychiatrist at Shizuoka Saiseikai General Hospital, Department of Psychiatry. The primary focus of his research is the electrophysiological analysis of attention and arousal in both humans and rodents. In clinical research, EEG, heart rate variability and skin conductance have been measured in mental disorders and arousal/consciousness disturbances. In basic research, single neuronal firing and EEG recordings have been assessed in rats. His research interests cover physiological rhythms related to attention, arousal, and consciousness in both the central and peripheral nervous systems, with a focus on understanding mental states.

Meet the Volume Editor

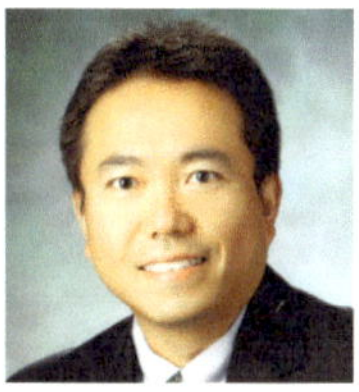

Liam Chen, MD, Ph.D., is a professor in the Department of Laboratory Medicine and Pathology at the University of Minnesota Medical School. Dr. Chen earned a Ph.D. in Genetics & Developmental Biology at the University of Alberta, Canada. After graduating, he received residence and fellowship training in Anatomic Pathology, Neuropathology, and Molecular Genetic Pathology at Harvard Medical School. Dr. Chen's research focuses on understanding the cellular and molecular biological pathways that lead to major central nervous system disorders. Dr. Chen has over 100 scholarly works, including research articles, reviews, and book chapters. He is a member of multiple editorial boards and grant evaluation and review bodies, including NIA/NIH, the Department of Defence, and the German Research Foundation.

Contents

Preface

This book brings together a comprehensive exploration of current advances in our understanding and management of multiple sclerosis (MS). Through a curated sequence of chapters, the book aims to bridge gaps in knowledge across genetics, environment, diagnostics, clinical presentation, and treatment strategies. Each chapter contributes a vital piece to the broader mosaic of MS research and care, offering insights for clinicians, researchers, and students alike.

We begin with *The Genetic and Environmental Determinants of Multiple Sclerosis: Unraveling the Complex Interactions in Disease Onset and Progression*, which sets the stage by examining how genetic predisposition and environmental exposures converge to influence the risk and course of MS. This foundational chapter establishes the multifactorial nature of the disease, highlighting key gene-environment interactions and their implications for prevention and early intervention. *Restoring Immune Balance in Multiple Sclerosis: The Impact of Skull Immunity* explores a novel frontier in neuroimmunology by examining the role of skull immunity in the pathogenesis and potential treatment of multiple sclerosis (MS). Traditionally, immune regulation in MS has focused on systemic and CNS-resident immune mechanisms. However, emerging research reveals that the skull bone marrow hosts a distinct population of immune cells that directly interact with the brain and meninges, thereby contributing uniquely to central nervous system (CNS) immune homeostasis. These interactions are increasingly recognized as pivotal in multiple sclerosis (MS), where dysregulation of immune activity leads to chronic central nervous system (CNS) inflammation and demyelination.

The following chapter, *Multi-Omics Profiling of Cerebrospinal Fluid: A Strategy for Unveiling Multiple Sclerosis*, delves into advanced diagnostic approaches. It presents the promise of multi-omics technologies, which integrate genomics, proteomics, metabolomics, and other fields to profile cerebrospinal fluid and detect biomarkers that can aid in earlier diagnosis and more personalized disease management. In *Atypical Presentation or Variants of Multiple Sclerosis*, the focus shifts to the clinical domain, concentrating on the diagnostic challenges presented by non-classical manifestations of MS. This chapter provides a detailed account of rare variants and unusual symptom patterns, emphasizing the need for nuanced clinical evaluation and tailored management strategies.

The integration of technology into clinical care is addressed in *Artificial Intelligence Algorithms in Neurology: Optimizing the Management of Patients with Multiple Sclerosis*. Here, the application of AI tools for diagnostic support, prognostic modeling, and treatment decision-making is explored, showcasing how machine learning can enhance precision and efficiency in MS management. Finally, the last two chapters, *When and How to Use Plasma Exchange Therapy for Difficult-to-Treat Multiple Sclerosis Patients* and *Cytoflavin in the Complex Therapy of Multiple Sclerosis*, focus on therapeutic strategies for managing refractory cases. These complementary discussions provide evidence-based guidance on the indications, timing, and procedural considerations for plasma exchange therapy and cytoflavin, underscoring their roles as valuable options in specific clinical scenarios.

Together, the chapters in this volume provide a comprehensive view of MS, spanning from molecular mechanisms to clinical practice, with an emphasis on innovation, complexity, and patient-centered care.

Liam Chen
Department of Laboratory Medicine and Pathology,
University of Minnesota Medical School,
Minneapolis, USA

Section 1

Mechanisms and Pathways

Chapter 1

The Genetic and Environmental Determinants of Multiple Sclerosis: Unraveling the Complex Interactions in Disease Onset and Progression

Esra Demir Unal

Abstract

Multiple sclerosis (MS) is a multifactorial progressive neurodegenerative disease in which both neurogenetic and neuroepidemiological precipitating factors play a role, and it is known that various environmental and hereditary parameters (geographic prevalence, hereditary recurrence risks, gender differences, and time-dependent changes in sex ratio) play a role in its etiology. Through genome sequencing projects, genome-wide association studies (GWAS) have facilitated the development and recognition of population-based catalogs of common genetic variations. More than 233 genetic loci have been unequivocally identified as being associated with multiple sclerosis (MS), more than 30 of which are related to the major histocompatibility complex (MHC). Many of these genetic variants are closely related to immunological and environmental processes along with epigenetic modifications and play a role in the induction of other systemic neurodegenerative and autoimmune diseases. The mechanisms explained for MS-related heredity and its epidemiological and environmental relationships are still insufficient. This section will discuss the determination of genetic and environmental factors contributing to the onset and progression of MS in the prodromal stages and their multifactorial interactions.

Keywords: environmental parameters, epigenetic modifications, genome-wide association studies (GWAS), major histocompatibility complex (MHC), multiple sclerosis, neurodegenerative disease, neuroepidemiology

1. Introduction

Multiple sclerosis (MS) is a demyelinating disease characterized by recurrent inflammation caused by inflammatory cells in the central nervous system and primarily affects young adults. The lifestyle, environmental, and genetic factors individuals possess during the prodromal stage—years before the clinical onset—may predispose them to disease progression. Understanding the intricate interactions between these factors is crucial for disease progression. While many contemporary treatments can delay disease progression, no definitive method to halt its course has yet been developed. Most modern therapies exert broad-spectrum effects on the immune system and are associated with significant side effect profiles. From this perspective, MS treatments continue to represent an unmet medical need. Therefore, a diagnostic model that integrates multidisciplinary approaches—including genetic, lifestyle, and environmental factors—could guide the development of therapeutic strategies and preventative measures. Although various genetic and environmental factors such as metabolic disorders, viral infections, and lifestyle habits (e.g., alcohol and smoking) have been associated with MS [1], research into the interactions between these environmental and genetic factors remains insufficient. Recent advances have provided significant insights into the genetic basis of susceptibility to MS. Notable developments include the discovery of the human leukocyte antigen (HLA) complex, a dense cluster of genes on the short arm of chromosome 6, and the application of genome-wide association studies (GWAS), which utilize large arrays of single nucleotide polymorphisms (SNPs) distributed throughout the genome. These methods have facilitated the identification of diverse genomic risk factors [2]. However, despite the known polygenic nature of MS, the precise mechanisms by which genetic susceptibility and environmental factors interact to drive disease onset and progression remain unclear.

In this section, we examine the determination of genetic and environmental factors thought to contribute to the initiation and progression of MS during the prodromal phase, as well as the interactions between these factors.

2. The genetic determinants of multiple sclerosis

The significance of ethnicity and family history in the etiopathogenesis of multiple sclerosis (MS) has gained increasing attention in recent years. Studies investigating the correlation between genetic predisposition and the risk of developing the disease have shown a marked rise in the past five decades. The relationship between ethnicity and MS has been examined in topographic properties, and countries with higher prevalence rates are observed in Scandinavia, Iceland, the British Isles, and North America (approximately 1–2 per 1000 individuals) [3]. In contrast, except in Sardinia, lower prevalence rates are observed in southern European populations. Among Asians, Amerindians, African Blacks, and the indigenous populations of New Zealand and Australia, MS is rarely reported.

Genetic investigations into the pathogenesis of MS have revealed that monozygotic twins have a higher concordance rate for MS (20–30%) compared to dizygotic twins of the same sex (2–5%). Additionally, siblings of individuals with MS are 10–15 times more likely to develop the disease than the general population, and increased prevalence has also been noted among second and third-degree relatives [4]. Besides this, recent GWAS attempts have provided empirical evidence supporting polygenic inheritance models involving allelic variants commonly associated with MS in the population [5]. The use of "SNP chips or arrays," designed to examine single nucleotide variations, has been instrumental in identifying hundreds of polymorphisms associated with various diseases, including MS. This progress instills confidence in the research community and paves the way for a deeper understanding of the genetic basis of MS and its related conditions.

In recent years, major histocompatibility complex (MHC) groups have emerged as significant genetic markers in the inheritance of MS. Genetic alterations within these complexes have been shown to influence the molecular basis of antigen presentation and alter the clinical course of both adult-onset MS (AOMS) and pediatric-onset MS (POMS). These findings provide the genetic foundation for autoimmune responses, where the body's immune system mistakenly attacks its own tissues, induced by environmental factors in the context of immunological synaptic connections in MS. Understanding this genetic foundation is crucial in comprehending the complex interplay between genetics and the environment in the development of MS [4].

In the last decades, there has been a marked increase in the incidence of MS, particularly among women [6]. This rise is thought to be heavily influenced by the interaction of genetic risk factors with environmental factors, which substantially contribute to the overall risk burden [7, 8]. The studies investigating the relationship between the risk of developing MS in monozygotic twins and the altitudinal characteristics of their birthplace have revealed that risk varies based on altitude. Higher concordance rates for MS have been observed among twins born in regions with higher MS prevalence [9]. Similar to many other neurodegenerative diseases, MS exhibits hereditary characteristics. Although the effect of any single predisposing variant is limited, multifaceted gene-gene (epistatic) and/or gene-environment interactions may significantly enhance the contribution of certain variants to overall genetic risk. These susceptibility genes can undergo epigenetic modifications, further complicating the inheritance of MS [10]. The role of environmental factors in this complex interplay cannot be overstated, as they can trigger or exacerbate the disease in genetically susceptible individuals.

2.1 HLA locus variants and their impact on MS susceptibility

MHC is located on the short arm of chromosome 6 at position 6p21, encompassing a 4.5 megabase region and containing over 200 genes. Many of the MHC-associated genes play critical roles in the development, maturation, and composition of the T-cell repertoire, as well as in regulating various immunological processes. HLA genes have been linked to a range of conditions, including infections, cancers, autoimmune diseases, and inflammatory disorders. HLA genes are classified into two main classes: Class I genes are encoded in the telomeric region, while Class II genes are encoded near the centromeric region. Both classes produce cell surface glycoproteins that present antigenic peptide fragments to T cells. Among these, HLA-DR, -DQ, and -DP molecules belong to Class II HLA and are expressed on the surface of antigen-presenting cells such as B cells, dendritic cells, and macrophages. These molecules function as receptors for peptides presented to $CD4^+$ T lymphocytes. A third gene group, Class III, whose existence has been recognized in recent years, is clustered between Class I and Class II regions. This group encodes complement proteins, 21-hydroxylase, tumor necrosis factor, and heat shock proteins. More than 10,000 alleles related to HLA Class I and Class II loci have been identified [11].

Although the association between multiple sclerosis (MS) and the major histocompatibility complex (MHC) was first reported approximately 50 years ago, research aimed at identifying the causative alleles and confirming whether antigen presentation is directly linked to MS risk remains in progress. Initial studies demonstrated associations with HLA Class I antigens A3 and B7, while subsequent research identified associations with HLA Class II polymorphisms Dw2 and DR2. To explain the observed allelic heterogeneity, at least two hypotheses have been proposed.

The first suggests a hierarchy of DRB1 allelotypes that directly influence MS risk to varying degrees, and the second posits the presence of another genetic variant located near all DRB1 haplotypes associated with MS. Studies on the relationship between MS and MHC alleles have highlighted the genetic predisposition and the association of specific alleles with particular HLA loci. HLA-DRB115:01 and HLA-DRB103:01 alleles have been reported to be associated with an increased risk of MS, whereas the HLA-A02:01 allele has been suggested to have a protective effect. Data from the Wellcome Trust Case Control Consortium (WTCCC) showed significant odds ratios (OR) for individuals carrying these alleles: HLA-DRB115:01 ($OR = 3.24$; $p < < 10^{-300}$), HLA-DRB103:01 ($OR = 1.27$; $p < 10^{-11}$), and HLA-A02:01 ($OR = 0.69$; $p < 10^{-53}$) [4, 12].

Most HLA alleles within the MHC region are tightly linked, forming a core collection across the HLA genes (HLA-A, HLA-C, HLA-B, HLA-DRB1, and HLA-DQB1) that spans at least 3 Mb of DNA. This core collection creates highly conserved extended haplotype regions (CEHs) [13]. These haplotypes are present across all human populations, and the Wellcome Trust Case Control Consortium (WTCCC) identified the 250 most common CEHs, predominantly in Europe, accounting for 57% of all CEHs [14, 15]. The tight linkage between HLA alleles is particularly pronounced between the HLA-DRB1 and HLA-DQB1 loci. In the WTCCC dataset, 97.5% of individuals with HLA-DRB115:01 (the most common DRB1 allele in Europe, with a control frequency of 13.0%) also carried HLA-DQB106:02. Similarly, 98.4% of HLA-DRB103:01 alleles (control frequency of 11.8%) were linked with HLA-DQB102:01. In another study, a novel SNP-haplotype collection spanning approximately 0.25 Mb of DNA in the HLA-DRB1 locus was identified, including SNPs such as rs2395173, rs2395174, rs3129871, rs7192, rs3129890, rs9268832, rs532098, rs17533090, rs2187668, rs1063355, and rs9275141 [16]. The Class II HLA-DRB103:01 ~ HLA-DQB102:01 haplotype has been categorized into two distinct forms: one (a6) linked with 84% of the WTCCC control group and another (a2) associated with 15% of the control group [14]. Studies have found a strong association between carrying the (H^+) haplotype and MS risk. While individuals without (H^+) who carry the (a2) haplotype may also be at risk for MS, those with the (a6) haplotype exhibit a risk gradient influenced by Class I regions, ranging from highly protective to highly risky [14, 15]. Although the (H^+) haplotype is linked to increased MS risk, this correlation may vary depending on the CEH. Similarly, certain HLA-DRB115:01 ~ HLA-DQB106:02 haplotypes lacking the (a1) SNP haplotype have not been associated with MS [14]. Other studies have demonstrated that although HLA-A*02:01 is protective against MS, some CEHs containing this allele exert little or no effect on MS susceptibility [15]. The strong linkage disequilibrium in the Class II region and the CEH structure of the MHC make it unclear which gene(s) are primarily responsible for MS risk [17].

While the interactions between genetic, geographic, and environmental factors contributing to MS remain incompletely understood, the MHC is the primary susceptibility locus for MS, with this relationship being particularly strong in MHC Class II. In a meta-analysis by Zhang et al., the DRB103 phenotype increased MS risk [16]. Romero et al. reported that DRB104 does not alter MS risk but negatively affects prognosis [18]. Another study found that DRB1*04 is more frequent in mestizo Mexican individuals [19]. A study investigated interactions between environmental factors and HLA genes, specifically HLA-DRB115:01 heterozygous and homozygous alleles. Participants were compared for MS risk concerning different genotypes, smoking status, EBNA-1 (Epstein-Barr Nuclear Antigen-1) status, and body mass index during adolescence. The findings indicated that the effect of HLA-DRB115:01 on MS risk follows an additive model on the log-odds scale. Moreover, the interaction between

HLA-DRB115:01 and environmental factors was similar in magnitude regardless of the allele count. However, in individuals carrying HLA-DRB115:01 without the protective HLA-A02:01 allele, exposure to environmental factors created a three-way interaction, resulting in a high odds ratio for MS. This risk was particularly elevated in homozygous carriers of HLA-DRB115:01 (e.g., smokers: OR = 20.0, 95% CI 13.1–30.5; individuals with high EBNA-1 antibody levels: OR = 21.9, 95% CI 15.0–31.8; adolescents reporting overweight/obesity: OR = 44.3, 95% CI 13.5–145) [20]. In a study involving the HLA-DRB104:03 genetic variant, the relationship between this genetic pattern and the response to disease-modifying therapy was investigated. It was reported that 86.7% of MS patients achieved NEDA-3, and no significant difference in the AA genetic variant was observed between patients who achieved NEDA-3 and those who did not (48.7 vs. 43.1%, $p = 0.6$) [21]. In a study conducted on non-Hispanic European MS patients, 11 HLA loci and 19 haplotype segments were genotyped using next-generation sequencing (NGS) [22]. The study revealed that the haplotypes DRB501:01:01 ~ DRB115:01:01:01 were significantly associated with MS susceptibility (gTDT: $p < 2.20e-16$; mTDT: $p = 1.61e-07$; CC: $p < 2.22e-16$), and the DRB115:01 haplotype was identified as an independent risk allele (gTDT: $p = 3.69e-03$; mTDT: $p = 2.99e-03$; CC: $p = 1.00e-02$). Additionally, the DRB101:01:01 allele was protective against MS (gTDT: $p = 8.68e-06$; mTDT: $p = 4.50e-03$; CC: $p = 1.96e-06$). Similarly, DQB1 alleles such as DQB103:01 (gTDT: $p = 2.86e-03$; mTDT: $p = 5.56e-02$; CC: $p = 4.08e-05$) and DQB103:03 (gTDT: $p = 1.17e-02$; mTDT: $p = 1.16e-02$; CC: $p = 1.21e-02$) demonstrated protective effects. Class I HLA alleles, including A02:0 1:01:01 ~ C03:04:01:01 ~ B40:01:02 (gTDT: $p = 5.86e-03$; mTDT: $p = 3.65e-02$; CC: $p = 9.69e-03$), B27:05 (gTDT: $p = 6.28e-04$; mTDT: $p = 2.15e-03$; CC: $p = 1.47e-02$), and B*38:01 (gTDT: $p = 3.20e-03$; mTDT: $p = 6.14e-03$; CC: $p = 1.70e-02$), were identified as moderately protective. Some studies suggested that HLA-associated MS risk might increase the risk of intracranial cancer [23]. An investigation across 14 Western European countries examining 127 high-resolution HLA alleles revealed a strong correlation between MS and brain cancer immunogenetic profiles ($p < 0.001$). This relationship was most prominent in DRB1, followed by DQB1 and HLA-A (26). Another study aimed to determine the association between HLA-DRB1 and HLA-DQB1 alleles and the IL7R (rs6897932) gene variant with MS. The prospective study demonstrated that HLA-DRB115:01/15:02 (OR = 3.65; $p < 0.0001$) and HLA-DQB106:02 (OR = 4.19, $p < 0.0001$) alleles were positively associated with MS, while HLA-DRB114:04:01 (OR = 0.21; $p = 0.0009$) showed a negative association. The haplotype with the strongest statistical association was HLA-DRB115:01-DQB1*06:02 (OR = 5.69, $p < 0.0001$) [24]. While the major histocompatibility complex (MHC) locus is recognized as having a dominant role in genetic susceptibility to MS, over 30 loci have been identified across various studies. In a study involving 161 MS patients, the impact of HLA alleles on T-cell receptor (TCR) CDR3 sequences was analyzed, identifying five MS risk loci: HLA-DRB115:01 ($p = 7.65 \times 10^{-3}$), rs9271366 ($p = 1.96 \times 10^{-3}$), rs766848979 A ($p = 1.89 \times 10^{-2}$), rs9277626 ($p = 2.95 \times 10^{-2}$), and rs11751659 ($p = 1.92 \times 10^{-2}$). Expanded clonotypes were identified in individuals with risk alleles, with specific associations observed for HLA-DRB115:01 ($p = 4.99 \times 10^{-3}$), rs9271366 ($p = 6.54 \times 10^{-3}$), rs1049079 C ($p = 4.37 \times 10^{-2}$), AA DQB1 position −5 L ($p = 1.05 \times 10^{-3}$), and AA DQB1 position 221 Q ($p = 9.39 \times 10^{-4}$) [25].

MS is primarily a chronic inflammatory disease of the central nervous system, where genetic predisposition is a critical determinant of disease risk. MHC-associated genes play pivotal roles in the development, maturation, and composition of the T-cell repertoire, as well as in regulating various immunological processes. These genes, categorized into HLA class I and II, have been associated with numerous infections, cancers, autoimmune diseases, and inflammatory conditions. The Wellcome Trust Case Control Consortium (WTCCC) dataset is one of the most comprehensive studies evaluating HLA alleles in MS risk. It identified HLA-DRB115:01 as the most strongly associated allele, along with other alleles such as HLA-DRB103:01 and HLA-A*02:01. The HLA region within the MHC locus comprises highly polymorphic genes and includes conserved extended haplotype regions (CEHs). According to WTCCC data, 250 CEHs have been identified. The haplotype formed by HLA-DRB115:01 and DQB106:02 significantly increases MS risk and is recognized as the strongest genetic risk factor for MS, while alleles such as HLA-DRB101:01 and HLA-DQB105:01 have demonstrated protective effects. Other alleles, including HLA-DQB1, HLA-DRB1, and HLA-DPB1, have contributed to MS risk in various configurations. Furthermore, the association of HLA alleles with TCR CDR3 sequence diversity has been implicated in forming MS risk loci.

2.2 Genome-wide association studies insights in MS susceptibility

The pathogenesis of multiple sclerosis (MS) involves a complex and multifactorial etiopathogenetic process encompassing genetic, environmental, and epigenetic factors. Genome-wide association studies (GWAS) are primarily used to investigate the relationship between genetic variations and specific diseases or phenotypes. By comparing the frequency of genetic variants between affected individuals and healthy controls, GWAS aims to identify factors contributing to disease susceptibility. In the context of MS, GWAS has significantly contributed to identifying genetic risk factors, understanding polygenic susceptibility, pinpointing risk genes and variants, identifying non-MHC risk genes, analyzing MS-associated regulatory regions, and examining the role of immune-specific cells in MS. The first GWAS on MS was conducted by the International Multiple Sclerosis Genetics Consortium (IMSGC), including 931 family trios (MS patients and their parents) and 2431 controls [26]. During the validation phase, an additional cohort of 609 independent family trios, 2322 MS cases, and 2987 controls was analyzed. For the first time, a non-MHC variant on chromosome 10p15, located in an intron of the interleukin-2 receptor alpha (IL2RA) gene, was identified as genome-wide significant in MS (p-value = 5×10^{-8}): rs12722489 ($p = 2.96 \times 10^{-8}$; OR = 1.25).

Additionally, a coding SNP on chromosome 5p13 in the interleukin-7 receptor alpha chain (IL7RA) gene, rs6897932 ($p = 2.94 \times 10^{-7}$; OR = 1.18), showed a similarly significant association. Subsequent studies expanded the number of genetic variants linked to MS [27–30]. In a cohort study involving 9772 European ancestry MS cases across 15 countries, IMSGC identified 49 MS-associated variants [31]. In later studies, IMSGC included other autoimmune diseases to identify common variants and developed the ImmunoChip (IC), a specialized genotyping array targeting approximately 200 regions and thousands of genome-wide genetic variants [32]. The project genotyped 14,498 MS cases and 24,091 controls, followed by validation in 14,802 MS cases and 26,703 controls. Ultimately, a list of 110 genome-wide significant variants was compiled. A larger cohort study of 14,802 MS cases and 26,703 controls conducted GWAS analysis, incorporating MS Chip data (20,360 MS cases and 19,047 controls) and ImmunoChip data (12,267 MS cases and 22,625 controls) in the validation phase [33]. This study identified 233 susceptibility variants with genome-wide significance, including 200 in the autosomal genome (outside the MHC region), 32 in the MHC region, and one on the X chromosome. The X chromosome association (rs2807267; OR = 1.07 for the T allele; p-value = 6.86×10^{-9}) was reported for the first time. Recent studies have focused on the heritability of MS, defined as the proportion of phenotypic variance explained by additive genetic effects. The total heritability for MS has been estimated at 19.2% [4], although most MS-associated genetic variants remain undiscovered. In a consortium study investigating the relationship between genetic variations and MS severity in 12,584 patients, the rs10191329 variant on chromosome 1p36.13 was found to be associated with disease severity. This variant was suggested to modulate MS by increasing the expression of the N-acetyltransferase 1 (NAT1) gene and affecting the central nervous system (CNS) resilience [34]. Another study integrated GWAS data with single-cell and bulk chromatin accessibility data and histone modification profiles to identify MS-associated genes and cell types. It demonstrated significant enrichment of MS-GWAS associations in regulatory regions of microglia and peripheral immune cell subtypes. Cell-specific polygenic risk scores were developed, allowing for the examination of correlations between MS risk, clinical phenotypes, and brain white matter volume [35]. A separate investigation of the interaction between genetic and epigenetic factors in MS compared genetic data from MS patients and healthy individuals. The findings suggested that epigenetic modifications significantly influence MS risk and may interact with genetic variants to influence disease progression [36].

GWAS studies have identified numerous genetic variants associated with MS, underscoring the importance of genetic contributions to the disease. Findings from GWAS suggest that most MS-associated genetic variations are related to the immune system, particularly involving microglia, T cells, B cells, and monocytes. These variations may influence transcriptional regulation, affecting gene expression and immune responses at the cellular level. Hypotheses suggest that these genetic variations could contribute to MS by altering immune response mechanisms, leading to autoimmune reactions against neural tissue, microglial activation, and brain inflammation. These processes may cause chromatin remodeling, resulting in aberrant gene expression in immune and neural cells. Identifying cellular-level interactions and their effects on the nervous system could provide hope and optimism for improved diagnosis and treatment.

2.3 Epigenetic modifications

Epigenetic mechanisms are biochemical processes that regulate gene expression without altering the underlying genetic sequence. These mechanisms are crucial in determining how cells read and utilize genetic information and mediating the interaction between genetic and environmental factors. Key epigenetic mechanisms identified to date include DNA methylation, histone modifications, non-coding RNAs, and chromatin remodeling.

Epigenetic processes facilitate the stabilization of biochemical changes across the genome, such as DNA methylation and post-translational modifications (PTMs), which regulate chromatin structure and transcription. For instance, genomic context determines the functional impacts of DNA modifications, such as gene expression regulation, stabilization, and X-chromosome inactivation. Methylation at CpG-rich promoter regions generally acts as a repressive signal, while DNA methylation within gene bodies can promote transcription [37, 38]. Active demethylation is mediated by the ten-eleven translocation (TET) protein family [39], which is highly expressed in brain tissue. The distinct role of 5-hydroxymethylcytosine (5hmC), derived from 5-methylcytosine (5mC), highlights its importance in neural tissues [40, 41]. Among PTMs, histone acetylation and methylation—regulated by histone acetyltransferases/deacetylases (HATs/HDACs) and methyltransferases/demethylases (e.g., HMTs/KDMs)—are particularly well-studied for their role in determining chromatin density and transcriptional activity [42].

Epigenetic processes are highly dynamic, occurring in cell-type-specific and developmental stage-specific contexts, and current research focuses on profiling these modifications across the genome. The first genome-wide study of DNA methylation differences in multiple sclerosis (MS) investigated the normal-appearing white matter (NAWM) from MS patients versus white matter (WM) from healthy controls [43]. Another study explored DNA methylation differences in demyelinated versus myelinated hippocampal tissues from MS patients [44]. A cell-specific analysis of subcortical white matter neurons in MS patients successfully distinguished methylation (5mC) from hydroxymethylation (5hmC) patterns [45]. An additional study examined the interaction between genetic risk factors, environmental exposures, and human leukocyte antigen (HLA) genes in MS. The interaction between HLA-DRB115:01 and environmental factors, independent of allele count, showed that HLA-DRB115:01 homozygosity combined with environmental exposure led to high odds ratios (ORs) due to triple interactions [20]. Using previously published DNA methylation (DNAm) datasets from case-control studies, epigenetic age acceleration (EAA) was calculated using whole blood DNAm data from 583 MS patients and 643 non-MS controls [46]. Results indicated increased EAA in MS patients compared to controls (~9 months, 95% CI: 3.6–14.4, $p = 0.001$). Moreover, EAA was found to be B-cell-dependent ($\beta int = 1.7$, 95% CI: 0.3–2.8, $p = 0.002$), with MS patients exhibiting a 5.1-year increase in EAA compared to controls (95% CI: 2.8–7.4, $p = 5.5 \times 10^{-5}$). Conversely, no EAA difference was observed in T-cell data. EAA was also associated with DNAm proxies for beta-2-microglobulin (difference = 47,546, 95% CI: 10,067–85,026; $p = 7.2 \times 10^{-5}$) and cigarette pack-years (difference = 8.1, 95% CI: 1.9–14.2, $p = 0.002$).

Emerging epigenetic evidence in MS suggests disrupted myelination balance and ongoing neuro-axonal damage contribute to disease progression. These alterations are closely linked to neuronal processes and may be influenced by internal factors, such as genetic variants, and external factors, such as smoking and aging. Epigenetic studies are essential for understanding the etiopathogenesis of MS and identifying molecular and cellular processes that could serve as targets for future therapeutic interventions.

3. The environmental determinants in multiple sclerosis

Multiple sclerosis (MS) is a progressive neurodegenerative and multifactorial disease influenced by immunogenetic factors and the interplay of various environmental risk factors. Numerous studies have proposed potential environmental triggers for MS. These include immutable factors such as ethnicity and gender, alongside modifiable factors like stress, obesity, vitamin deficiencies, dietary habits, trauma, tobacco use, sunlight exposure, cosmic rays, toxic exposures, occupational risks, and living with pets. Moreover, viral infections, particularly Epstein-Barr virus (EBV), human herpesvirus 6, and other viral strains like smallpox and varicella, have been implicated. While many environmental factors have been associated with MS, this section focuses on those with substantial evidence of involvement.

3.1 Gender and ethnicity

Gender differences are well-documented in autoimmune diseases, with women being more predisposed to autoimmune conditions than men [47, 48]. MS typically manifests in the second and third decades of life and is 2–3 times more prevalent in women, though it tends to follow a milder clinical course in females [49, 50]. The underlying etiopathogenesis suggests that women have a more dominant T-helper 1 (Th1) immune response than men, aligning with MS's Th1-driven activation pathways. This could explain the higher prevalence of MS in women [51, 52]. Hormonal processes and gender-associated genes are also hypothesized to influence MS development through interactions with neuroendocrine pathways. From a neuroendocrine perspective, estradiol, a subgroup of estrogen synthesized from cholesterol and acetyl-CoA through progesterone and testosterone intermediates, has been shown to increase IL-10 and IFN-γ production in CD4 T cells, suppressing T-cell-dependent inflammation [53]. However, since T cells lack estrogen receptors, estrogen's immunological effects are mediated through stromal cells, fibroblasts, and macrophages [54]. Low estrogen levels enhance the proinflammatory Th1 response, whereas high estrogen and progesterone levels promote a Th2 response. The decline in estrogen levels may trigger Th1-mediated inflammation, potentially exacerbating disease activity. In men, excessive activation of the hypothalamic-pituitary-adrenal axis, which reduces testosterone levels, has been linked to inflammation [55]. Testosterone is thought to play a protective role in remyelination, as supported by research findings [56]. Additionally, dehydroepiandrosterone (DHEA), a testosterone metabolite, has demonstrated anti-inflammatory properties, and some studies suggest that DHEA supplementation may yield beneficial outcomes in MS patients [57].

Studies exploring the relationship between MS prevalence and ethnicity have identified higher risks among White and Black individuals, while Hispanic and Asian populations exhibit lower prevalence rates. However, further research is required to determine whether MS susceptibility and prevalence vary among individuals from different cultural or ancestral backgrounds within these populations. A large-scale retrospective cohort study involving >2.6 million adults identified 3863 MS patients. The mean age of MS patients was 51.7 years (SD 13.1 years), and 76.8% were female. Women represented a higher proportion of Black (81.2%) and Asian (83.6%) MS patients compared to White (76.3%) or Hispanic (74.5%) individuals. Age and gender-standardized MS prevalence was similarly high among Black (95% CI: 207.1–244.5) and White (95% CI: 228.2–247.2) populations, while significantly lower in Hispanic (95% CI: 64.4–75.5) and Asian (95% CI: 17.1–28.1) populations. MS prevalence peaked across all racial and ethnic groups aged between 35 and 64 [58].

3.2 Smoking and tobacco use

A dose-response relationship between smoking and the risk of developing multiple sclerosis (MS) has been proposed, suggesting that cumulative smoking increases MS risk [59, 60]. Small-scale studies have reported an odds ratio (OR) of approximately 1.5 [61, 62], which was later confirmed by larger-scale case-control studies [59]. The detection of cotinine levels ≥10 ng/ml in the plasma of smokers prior to MS onset has contributed to the development of risk models for smoking [61]. Moreover, passive smoking exposure has also been linked to an increased risk of MS [62], possibly due to the slower onset of pulmonary damage in passive smokers. The primary causal relationship between smoking and MS has been hypothesized to arise from non-specific pulmonary damage, and similarly, exposure to organic solvents may act through a comparable pathway [63]. Smoking has also been associated with an increased risk of developing neutralizing antibodies against intravenous immunosuppressant drugs used in MS treatment, such as natalizumab and IFNβ [64].

Interestingly, in some cultures, tobacco is consumed orally in its pure form without the additives present in cigarettes. Unlike smoking, oral tobacco use has been reported to exhibit a dose-dependent inverse relationship with MS risk [65]. This has been attributed to nicotine modulating the α7 subunit of acetylcholine receptors in immune cells, thereby reducing receptor activity [66]. The increased risk associated with smoking may, therefore, stem from enhanced pulmonary inflammation. Smoking is believed to aggravate pulmonary inflammation, provoking proinflammatory pathways [67]. Central nervous system (CNS) autoantigenic cells in the lungs may activate in this hyperinflammatory environment and subsequently target the CNS. Experimental autoimmune encephalomyelitis (EAE) models have demonstrated the migration of encephalitogenic cells from the pulmonary region to the CNS [68].

Studies exploring the interaction between environmental factors and genetic predisposition have examined smoking in the context of human leukocyte antigen (HLA) variants. In Scandinavian populations, carrying the class II HLA-DRB115:01 MS risk allele has been associated with an OR of ~3, while the absence of HLA-A02 has been linked to an OR of ~1.8. Among non-smokers, a combined OR of ~5 has been reported, whereas smokers show a markedly increased combined OR of ~14 [69]. Similar results have been observed for passive smokers [70]. While no clear associations have been established between non-HLA genes and smoking, one interaction between a common non-HLA gene variant and smoking has been reported [71]. Smoking has been shown to interact with HLA class II variants, including HLA-DRB104 and HLA-DRB103 [72]. The proposed underlying mechanism suggests that smoking-induced hyperinflammatory environments facilitate the activation of CD4+ T cells, triggering autoimmune processes such as MS, rheumatoid arthritis, and polymyositis. Smoking may induce pulmonary enzymes, leading to post-translational modifications (e.g., citrullination) of peptides, thereby promoting the formation of peripheral autoimmune T cells and contributing to the onset of autoimmunity.

3.3 Epstein-Barr virus (EBV) and other viral agents exposure

While various infectious agents have been implicated in the etiology of multiple sclerosis (MS), the strongest evidence exists for Epstein-Barr virus (EBV). A meta-analysis [73] demonstrated that individuals with clinically symptomatic EBV infections have at least a twofold increased risk of developing MS. Another study found that individuals with MS exhibit higher titers of antibodies against EBV nuclear antigen 1 (EBNA1) and its epitope (amino acids 385–420) compared to healthy controls [74, 75]. One of the most striking findings involves EBNA1-negative individuals who seroconvert to EBNA1 antibody positivity prior to developing MS [76]. Studies indicate that the critical period for EBV exposure is during adolescence or later [77, 78]. The relationship between EBV and genetic risk appears to follow a pattern similar to smoking. Elevated anti-EBNA1 titers correlate positively with genetic predisposition to MS, and both infectious mononucleosis and increases in EBNA1 antibody titers have been associated with HLA risk variants for MS [79]. Among HLA variants, HLA-DRB1*15:01 shows the strongest association with EBV [80]. HLA risk alleles are hypothesized to encode molecules that modulate T-cell adaptive immunity in etiopathogenetic processes. Another hypothesis suggests that EBV persists latently within B cells, which are targeted by anti-CD20 therapies, making these treatments a significant option for MS management [81].

In contrast, cytomegalovirus (CMV) exposure (seropositivity) has been associated with a reduced risk of MS, with an odds ratio (OR) of ~0.7 in a case-control cohort study [82]. Furthermore, the rate of conversion to MS following the first clinical attack was reported to be lower among CMV-seropositive individuals compared to those who were CMV-seronegative [83]. The underlying etiopathogenetic mechanisms for this relationship remain unclear. A large-scale meta-analysis investigating the association between MS risk and other herpesvirus family members reviewed 289 datasets. It reported a combined prevalence of herpesvirus infections among individuals with MS as 50% (95% confidence interval [CI]: 45–55%; $I^2 = 96.91\%$). Subgroup analyses revealed combined prevalences for specific herpesviruses as follows: herpes simplex virus (HSV), 32%; varicella-zoster virus (VZV), 52%; EBV, 74%; CMV, 41%; human herpesvirus 6 (HHV-6), 39%; human herpesvirus 7 (HHV-7), 28%; and human herpesvirus 8 (HHV-8), 28%. These findings demonstrate a statistically significant correlation between human herpesvirus infections and MS risk, with a pooled OR of 2.07 (95% CI: 1.80–2.37; $I^2 = 80$) [84].

3.4 Vitamin D and sunlight exposure

A series of studies investigating the relationship between sunlight exposure, vitamin D levels, and MS risk gained prominence with the emergence of evidence linking MS incidence to latitudinal patterns. Numerous studies have suggested that ultraviolet radiation (UVR) and vitamin D protect against MS, demonstrating a significant inverse association between increased UV exposure and MS risk [85, 86]. However, the physiological mechanisms underlying this relationship remain unclear. In experimental autoimmune encephalomyelitis (EAE) models, UVR exposure has been shown to exert neuroprotective effects against inflammation, independent of vitamin D levels [87]. Additionally, UVR reduces peripheral inflammation [88]. The underlying mechanisms may involve UVR-induced activation of regulatory T cells (Tregs), resulting in modulatory effects on dendritic cells [89, 90]. This effect may be mediated through the induction of cis-urocanic acid production [91]. Munger et al. [92] reported that elevated vitamin D levels before the second decade of life might reduce MS risk in later decades.

Furthermore, concurrent sunlight exposure and a diet rich in omega-3 fatty acids could further decrease this risk [93]. Studies examining the effects of maternal vitamin D levels during pregnancy on MS risk in offspring have not identified significant differences between normal and affected individuals [94]. However, another study found that low maternal postpartum vitamin D levels within the first 3 months doubled the risk of MS in children [95]. Research on the relationship between vitamin D and genetic risk factors indicates that polymorphisms near the CYP27B1 gene, critical in vitamin D metabolism, increase MS risk [96]. Genetic factors influencing vitamin D levels significantly impact MS susceptibility [97]. The first gene-environment interaction identified in MS genetics involved vitamin D and the HLA DRB1*15:01 allele [98]. Despite extensive research, the roles of vitamin D levels and sunlight exposure in modulating MS risk remain contentious.

4. Gene-environment interactions

The multifaceted etiopathogenic processes underlying MS are shaped by interactions between genetic and environmental determinants, which play crucial roles in defining risk factors and influencing disease prognosis.

Attempts to model MS risk using polygenic risk scores (PRS) have focused on widespread genome-wide variants with a primary emphasis on MHC contributions. However, much of the risk for developing MS remains unexplained, leading to the hypothesis that genetic variants and environmental exposures may jointly create distinct risk models. Evidence from Scandinavian and North American cohorts suggests that environmental risk factors can be modified via HLA genotypes. For instance, early-life exposures to obesity, smoking, and certain solvents have been shown to increase MS risk in carriers of the HLA DRB115 allele and individuals lacking the protective HLA A02 genotype [99]. A study examining whether genetic risk factors alter the effects of environmental risks analyzed 2250 MS patients. The study found significant associations between MS and childhood obesity, early menarche, and smoking. Additionally, a strong interaction between childhood obesity and polygenic risk for MS was observed (PRSMHC: AP = 0.17, 95% CI 0.06–0.25, $p = 0.004$; PRSnon-MHC: AP = 0.17, 95% CI 0.06–0.27, $p = 0.006$) [100].

The interplay between genetic and environmental factors in MS remains incompletely understood. Risk models involving the joint interaction of these factors highlight the complexity of disentangling their relative contributions. Thus, assessing the independent importance of either genetic or environmental components may not yield meaningful scientific insights.

5. Conclusion

Multiple sclerosis (MS) is a complex and multifactorial progressive disease that leads to degenerative damage in the CNS. While its pathogenesis is not yet fully understood, it is widely accepted that genetic predisposition and environmental factors interact significantly to influence the disease's onset, progression, and severity. Genetic risk factors play a central role in the development of MS, with the most strongly associated genetic determinant being the HLA region. Studies have demonstrated a robust correlation between certain specific HLA alleles and increased MS risk. Genetic variants, particularly those that modulate the immune response of T and B cells, contribute to the disease's onset, and understanding how these genetic factors interact with environmental triggers is crucial to unraveling MS etiology. GWA studies provide an extensive strategy for uncovering the genetic basis of MS, aiming to identify genetic regions associated with the disease by examining numerous variants across the entire genome. These studies are pivotal in understanding how non-HLA genetic variants contribute to MS development. In addition to the genetic risk factors identified thus far, epigenetic factors are becoming increasingly recognized as important in understanding MS etiology. Epigenetic alterations, which regulate gene expression in response to environmental factors without altering the genetic structure, contribute to MS pathogenesis. DNA methylation, histone modifications, and changes in RNA levels can influence the immune system, thus increasing MS risk. Environmental triggers, such as toxic exposures and various viral strains, are known to be linked to an increased risk of MS. The complex interactions between these genetic and environmental triggers create a much more unpredictable and intricate environment for MS risk than the sum of their individual effects. These interactions influence disease progression, and both genetic and environmental factors play a role in accelerating or potentially mitigating the progression from the prodromal stage to the relapse stage. Furthermore, it is suggested that environmental factors, particularly viral infections and smoking, contribute to MS development via epigenetic mechanisms. Consequently, adopting a holistic approach to understanding the pathogenesis of the disease, including how it shapes its onset and progression, is crucial for developing targeted prevention strategies, early diagnostic tools, and personalized treatment methods.

Acknowledgements

All authors certify that they have no affiliations with or involvement in any organization or entity with any financial interest or non-financial interest in the subject matter or materials discussed in this manuscript.

Conflicts of interest

The authors have no potential conflicts of interest to disclose.

Notes/thanks/other declarations

This research did not receive any specific grant from funding agencies in the public, commercial, or not-for-profit sectors.

Author details

Esra Demir Unal
Ankara Yıldırım Beyazıt University, Medical Faculty Department of Neurology, Turkey

*Address all correspondence to: md.esrademir@gmail.com

References

[1] Alfredsson L, Olsson T. Lifestyle and environmental factors in multiple sclerosis. Cold Spring Harbor Perspectives in Medicine. 2019;**9**(4):a028944. DOI: 10.1101/cshperspect.a028944

[2] Olsson T, Barcellos LF, Alfredsson L. Interactions between genetic, lifestyle, and environmental risk factors for multiple sclerosis. Nature Reviews. Neurology. 2017;**13**(1):25-36. DOI: 10.1038/nrneurol.2016.187

[3] Sawcer S, Franklin RJ, Ban M. Multiple sclerosis genetics. The Lancet Neurology. 2014;**13**(7):700-709

[4] International Multiple Sclerosis Genetics Consortium (IMSGC). Multiple sclerosis genomic map implicates peripheral immune cells and microglia in susceptibility. Science. 2019;**365**(6460):eaav7188. DOI: 10.1126/science.aav7188

[5] Patsopoulos NA. Genetics of multiple sclerosis: An overview and new directions. Cold Spring Harbor Perspectives in Medicine. 2018;**8**(7):a028951. DOI: 10.1101/cshperspect.a028951

[6] Orton SM, Herrera BM, Yee IM, et al. Sex ratio of multiple sclerosis in Canada: A longitudinal study. Lancet Neurology. 2006;**5**:932-936

[7] Ascherio A, Munger KL. Environmental risk factors for multiple sclerosis. Part I: The role of infection. Annals of Neurology. 2007;**61**:288-299

[8] Ascherio A, Munger KL. Environmental risk factors for multiple sclerosis. Part II: Noninfectious factors. Annals of Neurology. 2007;**61**:504-513

[9] Islam T, Gauderman WJ, Cozen W, Hamilton AS, Burnett ME, Mack TM. Differential twin concordance for multiple sclerosis by latitude of birthplace. Annals of Neurology. 2006;**60**:56-64

[10] Otaegui D, Baranzini SE, Armananzas R, et al. Differential micro RNA expression in PBMC from multiple sclerosis patients. PLoS One. 2009;**4**:e6309

[11] Vandiedonck C, Knight JC. The human major histocompatibility complex as a paradigm in genomics research. Briefings in Functional Genomics & Proteomics. 2009;**8**:379-394

[12] Chao MJ, Barnardo MC, Lincoln MR, et al. HLA class I alleles tag HLA-DRB1*1501 haplotypes for differential risk in multiple sclerosis susceptibility. Proceedings of the National Academy of Sciences of the United States of America. 2008;**105**:13069-13074

[13] Lincoln MR, Ramagopalan SV, Chao MJ, et al. Epistasis among HLA-DRB1, HLA-DQA1, and HLA-DQB1 loci determines multiple sclerosis susceptibility. Proceedings of the National Academy of Sciences of the United States of America. 2009;**106**:7542-7547

[14] Goodin DS, Khankhanian P. Single nucleotide polymorphism (SNP)-strings: An alternative method for assessing genetic associations. PLoS One. 2014;**9**(4):e90034

[15] Goodin DS, Khankhanian P, Gourraud PA, Vince N. Highly conserved extended haplotypes of the major histocompatibility complex and their relationship to multiple

sclerosis susceptibility. PLoS One. 2018;**13**(2):e0190043

[16] Goodin DS, Khankhanian P, Gourraud PA, Vince N. Genetic susceptibility to multiple sclerosis: Interactions between conserved extended haplotypes of the MHC and other susceptibility regions. BMC Medical Genomics. 2021;**14**(1):183. DOI: 10.1186/s12920-021-01018-6

[17] Goodin DS, Khankhanian P, Gourraud PA, Vince N. The nature of genetic and environmental susceptibility to multiple sclerosis. PLoS One. 2020;**16**(3):e0246157

[18] Romero-Pinel L, Pujal JM, Martínez-Yélamos S, Gubieras L, Matas E, Bau L, et al. HLA-DRB1: Genetic susceptibility and disability progression in a Spanish multiple sclerosis population. European Journal of Neurology. 2011;**18**(2):337-342. DOI: 10.1111/j.1468-1331.2010.03148.x

[19] Vargas-Alarcón G, Gamboa R, Zuñiga J, Hernández-Pacheco G, Ramos-Kuri M, Castillo E, et al. HLA-DR4 allele frequencies on Indian and mestizo population from Mexico. Human Immunology. 2000;**61**(3):341-344. DOI: 10.1016/s0198-8859(99)00180-9

[20] Hedström AK, Hillert J, Brenner N, Butt J, Waterboer T, Strid P, et al. DRB1-environment interactions in multiple sclerosis etiology: Results from two Swedish case-control studies. Journal of Neurology, Neurosurgery, and Psychiatry. 2021;**92**(7):717-722. DOI: 10.1136/jnnp-2020-325676

[21] Gomez-Gaitan EA, Garcia-Ortega YE, Saldaña-Cruz AM, et al. Genetic variant HLA-DRB1*0403 and therapeutic response to disease-modifying therapies in multiple sclerosis: A case-control study. International Journal of Molecular Sciences. 2023;**24**(19):14594. DOI: 10.3390/ijms241914594

[22] Osoegawa K, Creary LE, Montero-Martín G, Mallempati KC, Gangavarapu S, Caillier SJ, et al. High resolution haplotype analyses of classical HLA genes in families with multiple sclerosis highlights the role of HLA-DP alleles in disease susceptibility. Frontiers in Immunology. 2021;**12**:644838. DOI: 10.3389/fimmu.2021.644838

[23] James LM, Georgopoulos AP. Positive association between the immunogenetic human leukocyte antigen (HLA) profiles of multiple sclerosis and brain cancer. Neuroscience Insights. 2023;**18**:26331055231214543. DOI: 10.1177/26331055231214543

[24] Vinoy N, Sheeja N, Kumar S, Biswas L. Class II HLA (DRB1, & DQB1) alleles and IL7R (rs6897932) variants and the risk for multiple sclerosis in Kerala, India. Multiple Sclerosis and Related Disorders. 2021;**50**:102848. DOI: 10.1016/j.msard.2021.102848

[25] Sorosina M, Santoro S, Ferrè L, Mascia E, Clarelli F, Giordano A, et al. Risk HLA variants affect the T-cell repertoire in multiple sclerosis. Neurology® Neuroimmunology & Neuroinflammation. 2023;**10**(3):e200093. DOI: 10.1212/NXI.0000000000200093

[26] International Multiple Sclerosis Genetics C, Hafler DA, Compston A, Sawcer S, Lander ES, Daly MJ, et al. Risk alleles for multiple sclerosis identified by a genomewide study. The New England Journal of Medicine. 2007;**357**:851-862

[27] Aulchenko YS, Hoppenbrouwers IA, Ramagopalan SV, Broer L, Jafari N, Hillert J, et al. Genetic variation in the KIF1B locus influences susceptibility

to multiple sclerosis. Nature Genetics. 2008;**40**:1402-1403

[28] Baranzini SE, Wang J, Gibson RA, Galwey N, Naegelin Y, Barkhof F, et al. Genome-wide association analysis of susceptibility and clinical phenotype in multiple sclerosis. Human Molecular Genetics. 2009;**18**:767-778

[29] De Jager PL, Jia X, Wang J, de Bakker PI, Ottoboni L, Aggarwal NT, et al. Meta-analysis of genome scans and replication identify CD6, IRF8, and TNFRSF1A as new multiple sclerosis susceptibility loci. Nature Genetics. 2009;**41**:776-782

[30] Jakkula E, Leppa V, Sulonen AM, Varilo T, Kallio S, Kemppinen A, et al. Genome-wide association study in a high-risk isolate for multiple sclerosis reveals associated variants in STAT3 gene. American Journal of Human Genetics. 2010;**86**:285-291

[31] International Multiple Sclerosis Genetics C, Wellcome Trust Case Control C, Sawcer S, Hellenthal G, Pirinen M, et al. Genetic risk and a primary role for cell-mediated immune mechanisms in multiple sclerosis. Nature. 2011;**476**:214-219

[32] International Multiple Sclerosis Genetics C, Beecham AH, Patsopoulos NA, Xifara DK, Davis MF, et al. Analysis of immune-related loci identifies 48 new susceptibility variants for multiple sclerosis. Nature Genetics. 2013;**45**:1353-1360

[33] Andlauer TF, Buck D, Antony G, Bayas A, Bechmann L, Berthele A, et al. Novel multiple sclerosis susceptibility loci implicated in epigenetic regulation. Science Advances. 2016;**2**(10):e1501678. DOI: 10.1126/sciadv.1501678

[34] International Multiple Sclerosis Genetics Consortium, Multiple MS Consortium. Locus for severity implicates CNS resilience in progression of multiple sclerosis. Nature. 2023;**619**(7969):323-331. DOI: 10.1038/s41586-023-06250-x

[35] Ma Q, Shams H, Didonna A, et al. Integration of epigenetic and genetic profiles identifies multiple sclerosis disease-critical cell types and genes. Communications Biology. 2023;**6**:342. DOI: 10.1038/s42003-023-04713-5

[36] Smith J et al. Investigation of genetic and epigenetic interactions in multiple sclerosis. Frontiers in Neurology. 2022;**13**:789. DOI: 10.3389/fneur.2022.00789

[37] Schubeler D. Function and information content of DNA methylation. Nature. 2015;**517**:321-326. DOI: 10.1038/nature14192

[38] Neri F, Rapelli S, Krepelova A, et al. Intragenic DNA methylation prevents spurious transcription initiation. Nature. 2017;**543**:72-77. DOI: 10.1038/nature21373

[39] Kriaucionis S, Tahiliani M. Expanding the epigenetic landscape: Novel modifications of cytosine in genomic DNA. Cold Spring Harbor Perspectives in Biology. 2014;**6**:a018630. DOI: 10.1101/cshperspect.a018630

[40] Mellen M, Ayata P, Dewell S, Kriaucionis S, Heintz N. MeCP2 binds to 5hmC enriched within active genes and accessible chromatin in the nervous system. Cell. 2012;**151**:1417-1430. DOI: 10.1016/j.cell.2012.11.022

[41] Lister R, Mukamel EA, Nery JR, et al. Global epigenomic reconfiguration during mammalian brain development. Science. 2013;**341**:1237905. DOI: 10.1126/science.1237905

[42] Strahl BD, Allis CD. The language of covalent histone modifications. Nature. 2000;**403**:41-45. DOI: 10.1038/35003126

[43] Huynh JL, Garg P, Thin TH, et al. Epigenome-wide differences in pathology-free regions of multiple sclerosis-affected brains. Nature Neuroscience. 2014;**17**:121-130. DOI: 10.1038/nn.3591

[44] Chomyk AM, Volsko C, Tripathi A, et al. DNA methylation in demyelinated multiple sclerosis hippocampus. Scientific Reports. 2017;**7**:8696. DOI: 10.1038/s41598-017-09537-2

[45] Kular L, Needhamsen M, Adzemovic MZ, et al. Neuronal methylome reveals CREB-associated neuro-axonal impairment in multiple sclerosis. Clinical Epigenetics. 2019;**11**:86. DOI: 10.1186/s13148-019-0678-x

[46] Maltby V, Xavier A, Ewing E, et al. Evaluation of cell-specific epigenetic age acceleration in people with multiple sclerosis. Neurology. 2023;**101**(7):e679-e689. DOI: 10.1212/WNL.0000000000207489

[47] Eidinger D, Garrett TJ. Studies of the regulatory effects of the sex hormones on antibody formation and stem cell differentiation. The Journal of Experimental Medicine. 1972;**136**:1098-1116. DOI: 10.1084/jem.136.5.1098

[48] Weinstein Y, Ran S, Segal S. Sex-associated differences in the regulation of immune responses controlled by the MHC of the mouse. Journal of Immunology. 1984;**132**:656-661

[49] Özakbaş S, İdiman E, Paköz B, Uysal U. Multipl sklerozda seyir özellikleri: 420 olgunun klinik özellikleri. Dokuz Eylül Üniversitesi Tıp Fakültesi Dergisi. 2003;**17**:205-211

[50] Miller A, Lublin F, Coyle PK. Multiple Sclerosis in Clinical Practice. 1st ed. CRC Press; 2003. DOI: 10.1201/9780367804442

[51] Kim S, Liva SM, Dalal MA, et al. Estriol ameliorates autoimmune demyelinating disease: Implications for multiple sclerosis. Neurology. 1999;**52**:1230-1238. DOI: 10.1212/WNL.52.6.1230

[52] Noseworthy JH, Lucchinetti C, Rodriguez M, Weinshenker BG. Multiple sclerosis. The New England Journal of Medicine. 2000;**343**:938-952. DOI: 10.1056/NEJM200009283431307

[53] Gilmore W, Weiner LP, Correale J. Effect of estradiol on cytokine secretion by proteolipid protein-specific T cell clones isolated from multiple sclerosis patients and normal control subjects. Journal of Immunology. 1997;**158**:446-451

[54] Villard-Mackintosh L, Vessey MP. Oral contraceptives and reproductive factors in multiple sclerosis incidence. Contraception. 1993;**47**:161-168. DOI: 10.1016/0010-7824(93)90135-L

[55] Wei T, Lightman SL. The neuroendocrine axis in patients with multiple sclerosis. Brain. 1997;**120**:1067-1076. DOI: 10.1093/brain/120.6.1067

[56] Dalal M, Kim S, Voskuhl RR. Testosterone therapy ameliorates experimental autoimmune encephalomyelitis and induces a T helper 2 bias in the autoantigen-specific T lymphocyte response. Journal of Immunology. 1997;**159**:3-6

[57] Roberts E, Fauble TJ. Oral DHEA in multiple sclerosis: Results of a phase one, open study. In: Kalimi M, Regelson W, editors. The Biologic Role

of DHEA. New York: Walter De Gruyter; 1990. pp. 81-93

[58] Langer-Gould AM, Gonzales EG, Smith JB, et al. Racial and ethnic disparities in multiple sclerosis prevalence. Neurology. 2022;**98**(18):e1818-e1827. DOI: 10.1212/WNL.0000000000200151

[59] Hedström AK, Baarnhielm M, Olsson T, Alfredsson L. Tobacco smoking, but not Swedish snuff use, increases the risk of multiple sclerosis. Neurology. 2009;**73**:696-701. DOI: 10.1212/WNL.0b013e3181b59c40

[60] Ghadirian P, Dadgostar B, Azani R, Maisonneuve P. A case-control study of the association between socio-demographic, lifestyle and medical history factors and multiple sclerosis. Canadian Journal of Public Health. 2001;**92**:281-285

[61] Hawkes CH. Smoking is a risk factor for multiple sclerosis: A meta-analysis. Multiple Sclerosis. 2007;**13**:610-615. DOI: 10.1177/1352458506073568

[62] Hedström AK, Hillert J, Olsson T, Alfredsson L. Exposure to environmental tobacco smoke is associated with increased risk for multiple sclerosis. Multiple Sclerosis. 2011;**17**:788-793. DOI: 10.1177/1352458510391537

[63] Barragan-Martinez C et al. Organic solvents as a risk factor for autoimmune diseases: A systematic review and meta-analysis. PLoS One. 2012;**7**:e51506. DOI: 10.1371/journal.pone.0051506

[64] Hedström AK, Hillert J, Olsson T, Alfredsson L. Smokers run increased risk of developing anti-natalizumab antibodies. Multiple Sclerosis. 2013;**20**:1081-1085. DOI: 10.1177/1352458513511197

[65] Hedström AK, Hillert J, Olsson T, Alfredsson L. Nicotine might have a protective effect in the etiology of multiple sclerosis. Multiple Sclerosis. 2013;**19**:1009-1013. DOI: 10.1177/1352458512471879

[66] Nizri E et al. Activation of the cholinergic anti-inflammatory system by nicotine attenuates neuroinflammation via suppression of TH1 and TH17 responses. Journal of Immunology. 2009;**183**:6681-6688. DOI: 10.4049/jimmunol.0902492

[67] Shan M et al. Lung myeloid dendritic cells coordinately induce TH1 and TH17 responses in human emphysema. Science Translational Medicine. 2009;**1**(4):4ra10. DOI: 10.1126/scitranslmed.3000116

[68] Odoardi F et al. T cells become licensed in the lung to enter the central nervous system. Nature. 2012;**488**:675-679. DOI: 10.1038/nature11337

[69] Hedström AK et al. Smoking and two human leukocyte antigen genes interact to increase the risk for multiple sclerosis. Brain. 2011;**134**:653-664. DOI: 10.1093/brain/awq371

[70] Hedström AK et al. Interaction between passive smoking and two HLA genes with regard to multiple sclerosis risk. International Journal of Epidemiology. 2014;**43**:1791-1798. DOI: 10.1093/ije/dyu155

[71] Briggs FB et al. Smoking and risk of multiple sclerosis: Evidence of modification by NAT1 variants. Epidemiology. 2014;**25**:605-614. DOI: 10.1097/EDE.0000000000000114

[72] Hedström AK, Rönnelid J, Klareskog L, Alfredsson L. Complex relationships of smoking, HLA-DRB1 genes, and serologic profiles in patients with early rheumatoid arthritis: Update

from a Swedish population-based case-control study. Arthritis & Rhematology. 2019;**71**(9):1504-1511. DOI: 10.1002/art.40852

[73] Handel AE, Giovannoni G, Ebers GC, Ramagopalan SV. An updated meta-analysis of risk of multiple sclerosis following infectious mononucleosis. PLoS One. 2010;**5**(9):e12496. DOI: 10.1371/journal.pone.0012496

[74] Sundström P, Nyström M, Ruuth K, Lundgren E. Antibodies to specific EBNA-1 domains and HLA DRB1*1501 interact as risk factors for multiple sclerosis. Journal of Neuroimmunology. 2009;**215**(1-2):102-107. DOI: 10.1016/j.jneuroim.2009.08.004

[75] Sundqvist E, Sundstrom P, Lindén M, Hedstrom AK, Alfredsson L, Hillert J, et al. Epstein-Barr virus and multiple sclerosis: Interaction with HLA. Genes & Immunity. 2012;**13**(1):14-20. DOI: 10.1038/gene.2011.47

[76] Levin LI, Munger KL, O'Reilly EJ, Falk KI, Ascherio A. Primary infection with the Epstein-Barr virus and risk of multiple sclerosis. Annals of Neurology. 2010;**67**(6):824-830. DOI: 10.1002/ana.21978

[77] Ascherio A, Munger KL. Epstein-Barr virus and autoimmunity. Current Topics in Microbiology and Immunology. 2015;**390**:365-385. DOI: 10.1007/978-3-319-22822-8_17

[78] Makhani N, Banwell B, Tellier R, Yeung R, Laughlin S, Konzak G, et al. Viral exposures and multiple sclerosis outcomes in a prospective cohort of children with acquired demyelination. Multiple Sclerosis. 2016;**22**(3):385-388. DOI: 10.1177/1352458515594043

[79] Zhou Y, Zhu G, Charlesworth J, Simpson S, Rubicz R, Mackay A, et al. Genetic loci for Epstein-Barr virus nuclear antigen-1 are associated with risk of multiple sclerosis. Multiple Sclerosis. 2016;**22**(7):889-899. DOI: 10.1177/1352458515598013

[80] Nielsen TR, Rostgaard K, Rasmussen S, Koch-Henriksen N, Haahr S. Effects of infectious mononucleosis and HLA DRB1*15 in multiple sclerosis. Multiple Sclerosis. 2009;**15**(4):431-436. DOI: 10.1177/1352458508100845

[81] Hauser SL, Waubant E, Arnold DL, Vollmer T, Antel J, Fox RJ, et al. B-cell depletion with rituximab in relapsing-remitting multiple sclerosis. New England Journal of Medicine. 2008;**358**(7):676-688. DOI: 10.1056/NEJMoa0706383

[82] Sundqvist E, Hillert J, Nystrom M, Sundstrom P. Cytomegalovirus seropositivity is negatively associated with multiple sclerosis. Multiple Sclerosis. 2014;**20**(2):165-173. DOI: 10.1177/1352458513490544

[83] Perri V, Zingaropoli MA, Pasculli P, Ciccone F, Tartaglia M, Baione V, et al. The impact of cytomegalovirus infection on natural killer and CD8+ T cell phenotype in multiple sclerosis. Biology. 2024;**13**(3):154. DOI: 10.3390/biology13030154

[84] Khalesi Z, Tamrchi V, Razizadeh MH, Letafati A, Moradi P, Habibi A, et al. Association between human herpesviruses and multiple sclerosis: A systematic review and meta-analysis. Microbial Pathogenesis. 2023;**177**:106031. DOI: 10.1016/j.micpath.2023.106031

[85] Kampman MT, Wilsgaard T, Mellgren SI. Outdoor activities and diet in childhood and adolescence relate to MS risk above the Arctic circle. Journal

of Neurology. 2007;**254**(4):471-477. DOI: 10.1007/s00415-006-0395-0

[86] Baarnhielm M, Hedström AK, Kockum I, Sundqvist E, Olsson T, Alfredsson L, et al. Sunlight is associated with decreased multiple sclerosis risk: No interaction with human leukocyte antigen-DRB1*15. European Journal of Neurology. 2012;**19**(8):955-962. DOI: 10.1111/j.1468-1331.2011.03650.x

[87] Becklund BR, Severson KS, Vang SV, DeLuca HF. UV radiation suppresses experimental autoimmune encephalomyelitis independent of vitamin D production. Proceedings of the National Academy of Sciences of the United States of America. 2010;**107**(14):6418-6423. DOI: 10.1073/pnas.1001119107

[88] Rana S, Rogers LJ, Halliday GM. Systemic low-dose UVB inhibits CD8 T cells and skin inflammation by alternative and novel mechanisms. American Journal of Pathology. 2011;**178**(6):2783-2791. DOI: 10.1016/j.ajpath.2011.02.045

[89] Breuer J, Schwab N, Schneider-Hohendorf T, Marziniak M, Mohan H, Bhatia U, et al. Ultraviolet B light attenuates the systemic immune response in central nervous system autoimmunity. Annals of Neurology. 2014;**75**(5):739-758. DOI: 10.1002/ana.24156

[90] Navid F, Kolbinger A, Zigrino P, Lichti J, Breitling T, Schwarz T, et al. The aryl hydrocarbon receptor is involved in UVR-induced immunosuppression. Journal of Investigative Dermatology. 2013;**133**(11):2763-2770. DOI: 10.1038/jid.2013.241

[91] Correale J, Farez MF. Modulation of multiple sclerosis by sunlight exposure: Role of cis-urocanic acid. Journal of Neuroimmunology. 2013;**261**(1-2):134-140. DOI: 10.1016/j.jneuroim.2013.05.005

[92] Munger KL, Levin LI, Hollis BW, Howard NS, Ascherio A. Serum 25-hydroxyvitamin D levels and risk of multiple sclerosis. Journal of the American Medical Association. 2006;**296**(23):2832-2838. DOI: 10.1001/jama.296.23.2832

[93] Cortese M, Riise T, Bjørnevik K, Holmøy T, Kampman MT, Magalhães S, et al. Timing of use of cod liver oil, a vitamin D source, and multiple sclerosis risk: The EnvIMS study. Multiple Sclerosis. 2015;**21**(14):1856-1864. DOI: 10.1177/1352458515579446

[94] Ueda P, Rafatnia F, Brännström T, Martin C, Alfredsson L, Wiberg M, et al. Neonatal vitamin D status and risk of multiple sclerosis. Annals of Neurology. 2014;**76**(3):338-346. DOI: 10.1002/ana.24210

[95] Munger KL, Åivo J, Hongell K, Soilu-Hänninen M, Surcel HM, Ascherio A. Vitamin D status during pregnancy and risk of multiple sclerosis in offspring of women in the Finnish maternity cohort. JAMA Neurology. 2016;**73**(5):515-519. DOI: 10.1001/jamaneurol.2015.4800

[96] Sundqvist E, Sundström P, Linden M, Hedström AK, Åivo J, Hillert J, et al. Confirmation of association between multiple sclerosis and CYP27B1. European Journal of Human Genetics. 2010;**18**(11):1349-1352. DOI: 10.1038/ejhg.2010.120

[97] Mokry LE, Ross S, Ahmad OS, Forgetta V, Smith GD, Goltzman D, et al. Vitamin D and risk of multiple sclerosis: A Mendelian randomization study. PLoS Medicine. 2015;**12**(8):e1001866. DOI: 10.1371/journal.pmed.1001866

[98] Handunnetthi L, Ramagopalan SV, Ebers GC. Multiple sclerosis, vitamin D, and HLA DRB1*15. Neurology. 2010;**74**(23):1905-1910. DOI: 10.1212/WNL.0b013e3181e24124

[99] Hedstrom AK, Hössjer O, Katsoulis M, Kockum I, Olsson T, Alfredsson L. Organic solvents and MS susceptibility: Interaction with MS risk HLA genes. Neurology. 2018;**91**(15):e455-e462

[100] Jacobs BM, Noyce AJ, Bestwick J, Belete D, Giovannoni G, Dobson R. Gene-environment interactions in multiple sclerosis: A UK biobank study. Neurology® Neuroimmunology & Neuroinflammation. 2021;**8**(4):e1007. DOI: 10.1212/NXI.0000000000001007

Chapter 2

Restoring Immune Balance in Multiple Sclerosis: The Impact of Skull Immunity

Yawei Liu, Xinchen Nie and Henrik Hasseldam

Abstract

Multiple sclerosis (MS) is a chronic autoimmune disorder characterized by immune-mediated damage to the central nervous system (CNS). Recent research highlights an emerging and intriguing area of investigation, "skull immunity," which refers to the unique immune cells within the skull bone marrow that directly interact with the CNS. Unlike peripheral bone marrow, skull immunity is specialized in regulating CNS immune homeostasis. The skull-derived immune response, alongside the glymphatic system and meningeal immunity, appears to significantly influence neuroinflammatory conditions such as MS. This expanding understanding of skull immunity adds complexity to our knowledge of CNS immunity and its role in MS pathogenesis. This chapter explores skull-derived immune responses, their interplay with the glymphatic system and meningeal immunity, and their specific contributions to neuroinflammatory processes. A deeper understanding of these mechanisms offers new opportunities for targeted therapies to restore immune balance and mitigate disease progression in MS.

Keywords: multiple sclerosis, T-cells, B-cells, skull immunity, autoimmunity

1. Introduction

Historically, the CNS was considered an immune-privileged organ due to the presence of the blood-brain barrier (BBB) and the absence of conventional lymphatic drainage [1]. This view suggested that the CNS was largely isolated from systemic immune activity, with minimal interactions between the peripheral immune system and CNS compartments. However, recent discoveries have overturned this traditional perspective, revealing that the CNS is dynamically connected to the immune system through various mechanisms, including specialized bone marrow niches [2, 3], meningeal lymphatic vessels [4–7], and cerebrospinal fluid (CSF) pathways [8–10]. These findings have profound implications for our understanding of multiple sclerosis (MS) and other neuroinflammatory conditions, as they highlight the role of peripheral and local immune systems in driving CNS inflammation.

IntechOpen

MS is a chronic inflammatory disease of the CNS characterized pathologically by demyelination, gliosis, neuro-axonal damage, and inflammation. Despite intense research, the precise mechanisms underlying the autoimmune attack on the CNS remain an active area of study [4, 9, 11–16]. One emerging area of investigation is the role of skull immunity—a concept that highlights the interactions between the CNS and bone marrow niches in the skull and vertebrae. Within these immune hubs, immune cells can directly communicate with the CNS through specialized channels. The proximity of skull bone marrow to the brain and the presence of channels connecting the skull marrow with the meninges (the protective layers around the brain) allow for direct interaction between skull-derived immune cells and the CNS, potentially enabling a rapid and localized immune response to CNS events. Therefore, skull immunity is now recognized as a crucial player in modulating neuroinflammatory responses in health and disease [2, 3, 17–20].

In this chapter, we would like to focus on:

1. CNS compartments are connected by their unique lymph circulation

2. CSF is involved in immune regulation in health and MS

3. Meningeal immunity in health and MS

4. Skull bone marrow in health and MS

5. Unanswered questions

6. Conclusions.

2. CNS compartments are connected by their unique lymph circulation

The CNS is responsible for monitoring and coordinating internal organ function while responding to environmental changes [21]. As a vital and highly specialized system, the CNS requires robust protection from both endogenous and exogenous threats, achieved through unique physical barriers and immune mechanisms.

In the mid-twentieth century, research introduced the concept of the CNS as an immune-privileged site, emphasizing its isolation from systemic immune processes. This idea was rooted in several unique characteristics of the CNS [22]. A key feature is the BBB, a highly selective physical and functional barrier. The BBB restricts the entry of pathogens, immune cells, and blood-derived factors through tight junctions between brain endothelial cells, the basal lamina, and astrocytic endfeet processes [23–26]. Additionally, the CNS lacks professional antigen-presenting cells (APCs) and exhibits low expression of MHC class I and II molecules in the brain parenchyma, further limiting immune surveillance. Furthermore, early studies suggested the absence of classical lymphatic vessels in the CNS, leading to the belief that CNS-derived antigens did not drain into peripheral lymph nodes. These characteristics were thought to contribute to the CNS's slow immune responses and limited interaction with the systemic immune system. Despite this perceived isolation, subsequent research has demonstrated significant interactions between the CNS and the immune system under both normal and pathological conditions. Immune privilege is now understood as a dynamic property, evolving as our understanding of neuroimmune interactions expands.

One early explanation for the CNS's immune privilege was the supposed absence of classical lymphatic drainage. However, recent evidence reveals that the CNS employs alternative drainage pathways for CSF and interstitial fluid (ISF) [27, 28], both critical for immune surveillance and homeostasis.

2.1 Drainage pathways of the CNS

- CSF is primarily produced by the choroid plexus in the brain's ventricles and circulates through the lateral ventricles, the third and fourth ventricles, and into the subarachnoid space. CSF drains into cervical lymph nodes (CLNs) via specialized channels passing through the cribriform plate of the ethmoid bone into the nasal mucosa. Antigen-presenting cells (APCs) migrate along these pathways, facilitating immune surveillance and interactions with the systemic immune system.

- ISF circulates within the brain parenchyma and drains through unique routes along the basement membranes of cerebral capillaries and arteries. These 100–150 nm-wide channels efficiently transport solutes and antigens to cervical lymph nodes, enabling antigen presentation and immune cell migration.

Unlike other organs, the CNS lacks conventional lymphatic vessels, but several well-defined pathways for the egress of cells and antigens from the brain have been identified [29, 30]. One of these specialized systems is the *glymphatic system*, which functions as a waste-clearance mechanism for the brain [31]. The glymphatic system operates by driving CSF flow from the subarachnoid space along perivascular spaces (PVS) surrounding penetrating arteries. This influx of CSF into the brain interstitium is facilitated by the astroglial water channel *aquaporin-4 (AQP4)*, predominantly expressed at the end feet of astrocytes lining the PVS [32]. Through this mechanism, CSF mixes with ISF, promoting a bulk flow of ISF that exits along perivenous spaces. This process is crucial for removing harmful proteins, metabolic byproducts, and other waste materials from brain tissue [33]. A schematic representation of this process is shown in **Figure 1**.

In the context of *MS*, the relationship between the glymphatic system and disease pathology appears to be bidirectional. MS-related inflammation may disrupt glymphatic system activity, impairing waste clearance and exacerbating neuroinflammation. For example, in animal models of MS, the reduction of spinal cord parenchymal CSF circulation was observed in experimental mice [34]. Similar observations were discovered in a human study, and Schubert et al. used dynamic ^{11}C-PiB PET *(11C-Pittsburgh compound B (PIB)-positron emission tomography)* to identify changes in CSF clearance and demonstrated deficits in ventricular CSF clearance in MS patients compared to healthy individuals [35]. Conversely, dysfunction of the glymphatic system could intensify MS symptoms by allowing the accumulation of harmful substances, such as proinflammatory molecules and protein aggregates, further aggravating disease progression [31]. For example, patients with MS generally had impaired glymphatic function compared to healthy controls, with more pronounced impairment seen in those with primary progressive MS (PPMS) as opposed to relapsing-remission MS (RRMS) [36]. Several factors may contribute to the interaction between the glymphatic system and MS progression. The glymphatic system is most active during slow-wave sleep, facilitated by reduced noradrenaline levels [37], and Buratti et al. explored the relationship between sleep quality and MS progression,

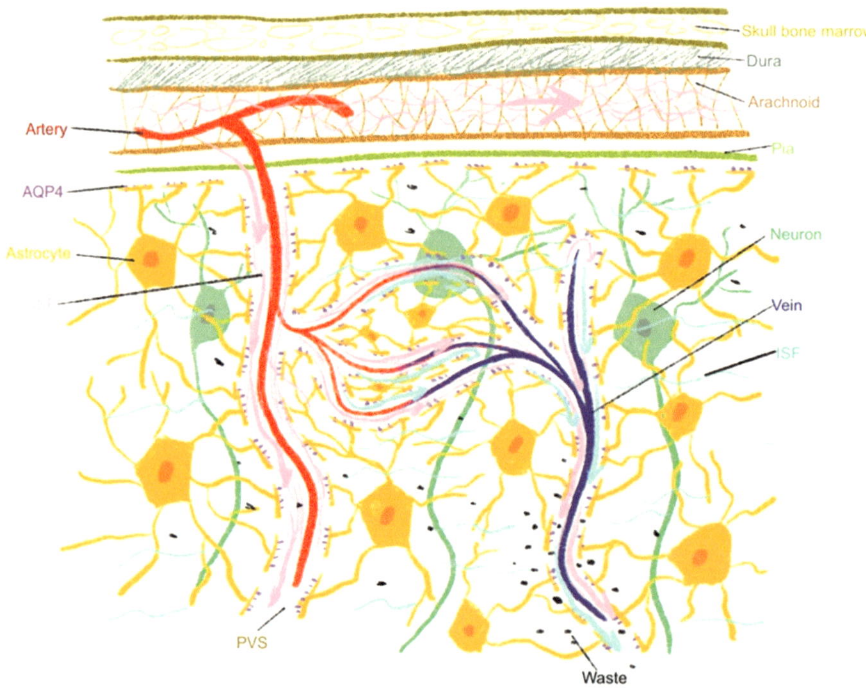

Figure 1.
Overview of the glymphatic system in the brain. The glymphatic system facilitates cerebrospinal fluid (CSF) (pink) movement from the subarachnoid space into the brain via perivascular spaces (PVS) surrounding penetrating arteries (red). This influx of CSF is driven by aquaporin-4 (AQP4) water channels (purple), which are predominantly localized on the end feet of astrocytes (yellow) lining the PVS. Once inside the brain, CSF mixes with interstitial fluid (ISF) (light blue), generating a bulk flow that exits along perivenous spaces. This process is vital in clearing metabolic waste, harmful proteins, and other byproducts (black) from brain tissue.

observing that patients with RRMS who experienced poor sleep had an increased rate of prolonged relapses over a month-long period [38]. Sleep disturbances not only impair glymphatic function but also exacerbate existing MS symptoms [31].

Additionally, disruptions in glymphatic function may be linked to altered AQP-4 expression [39], perivascular space impairment [40], or dysfunction in meningeal lymphatic vessels [41]. These impairments can potentially result in the accumulation of inflammatory and neurotoxic substances, further impacting the glymphatic system and contributing to neuroinflammation. While connections between glymphatic dysfunction, MS, and related factors are becoming more evident, further research is required to elucidate the precise mechanisms and their potential therapeutic implications in more detail [31].

As the glymphatic system drains the immune cells from the CSF into the cervical lymph nodes (CLNs) [42], CLNs exhibit unique properties for inducing immune tolerance [43]. Studies have shown that removing CLNs reduces lesion and disease load in experimental autoimmune encephalomyelitis (EAE), an animal model of multiple sclerosis (MS) [44, 45]. Similarly, lumbar lymph nodes, which drain the spinal cord, are implicated in regulating spinal inflammation, further underscoring their relevance as potential therapeutic targets for CNS diseases [46, 47]. Despite the absence of conventional lymphatics, the efficient drainage of both CSF and ISF to regional lymph nodes allows for immune cell migration, antigen presentation, and systemic immune interactions. These mechanisms are critical in neuroinflammatory conditions like MS, where targeting cervical and lumbar lymph nodes could enhance immune regulation and potentially improve therapeutic outcomes.

The CNS, long thought to be isolated from the immune system, employs highly specialized drainage pathways that integrate neuroimmune interactions with systemic immunity. The evolving understanding of CNS drainage mechanisms has profound implications for developing innovative therapies in modulating the lymphatic drainage pathways, immune cell migration, or antigen presentation for the treatment of CNS diseases. These mechanisms are central to maintaining immune homeostasis under physiological conditions and driving immune responses during pathology.

3. CSF is involved in immune regulation in health and MS

CSF is a plasma-like liquid essential for brain homeostasis, playing critical roles in *nutrient delivery, waste removal, and mechanical protection*. Produced primarily by the *choroid plexus* located in the lateral, third, and fourth ventricles, a smaller portion of CSF is secreted by the *ependymal cells* lining the ventricles. After its production, CSF circulates through the ventricular system, enters the subarachnoid space, and is eventually reabsorbed into venous circulation via *arachnoid villi* [48]. Importantly, the CSF functions as a key component of the *glymphatic system*, a waste-clearance mechanism in which brain-derived molecules are cleared via CSF efflux to the parasagittal dura mater and drained through meningeal lymphatic vessels. This pathway facilitates immune surveillance of the CNS from peripheral sites [49, 50]. Recent evidence also highlights that CSF can access skull bone marrow niches, regulating *myelopoiesis* and the subsequent egress of myeloid cells to the meninges under both physiological and pathological conditions [17]. This process is explained in **Figure 2**.

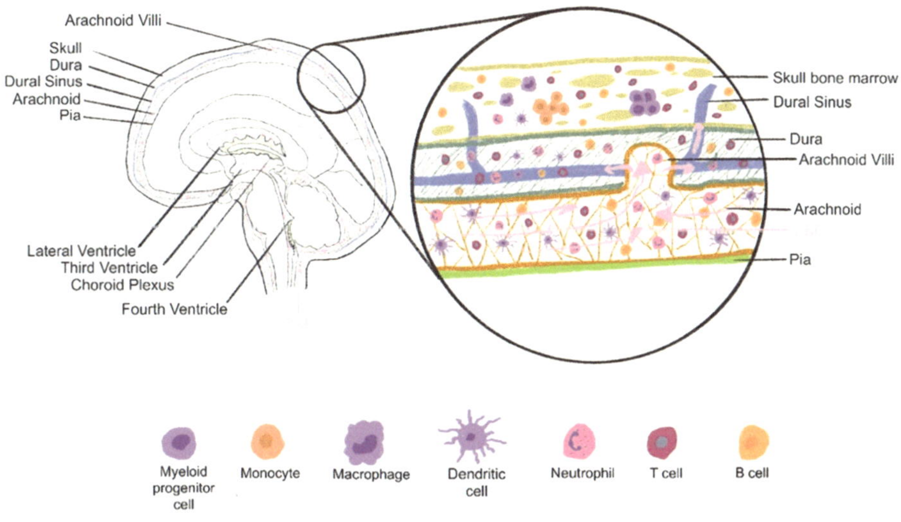

Figure 2.
CSF in CNS immunity. Left: the overview of cerebrospinal fluid (CSF) (pink) production and circulation. CSF is mainly produced by the choroid plexus (green) in the brain's ventricles, with a smaller contribution from ependymal cells lining the ventricles. CSF flows through the ventricular system, enters the subarachnoid space, and is reabsorbed into venous circulation via arachnoid villi. Right: the enlarged region with arachnoid villi and cellular composition in the skull and meninges. After CSF is absorbed by arachnoid villi, it drains to the dural venous sinuses and meningeal lymphatic vessels, enabling immune surveillance.

CSF hosts a tightly regulated immune environment, which maintains CNS homeostasis. Recent advancements in *single-cell transcriptomic analyses* have revealed compartment-specific immune cell compositions and highlighted how they change during neuroinflammation. In healthy individuals, the majority of immune cells in CSF are *CD4+ T cells*, comprising approximately *50%* of the immune cell population, while *CD8+ T cells* account for around *18%*. In contrast, B cells and monocytes are less abundant [51]. During neuroinflammation, as observed in MS, the immune composition of the CSF undergoes substantial alterations. Compared to peripheral blood, the CSF demonstrates a notable enrichment of myeloid dendritic cells (mDC), which play a key role in antigen presentation and immune modulation. Additionally, monocytes within the CSF exhibit distinct transcriptional profiles that closely resemble CNS border-associated macrophages, highlighting their potential specialization in responding to neuroinflammatory conditions [52]. Furthermore, both *CD4+ T cells* and Tregs are found in higher abundance in CSF compared to peripheral blood [53]. Among the altered CD4+ T cell populations in MS, *cytotoxic CD4+ T cells* have been of particular interest. These cells exhibit an expanded phenotype in MS-derived CSF and are thought to locally contribute to CNS pathology [54]. These findings collectively emphasize that specific immune cell populations—particularly CD4+ T cells with cytotoxic properties—play an active role in promoting local inflammation in MS.

Given the intimate relationship between *T cells* and *B cells* in MS pathogenesis, it is hypothesized that *pathological interactions* between *T follicular helper (TFH) cells* and B cells in the CSF locally drive autoimmune reactions [55]. Supporting this hypothesis, studies have shown the *expansion of B cell clones* in the CSF of MS patients [56] partially due to migration from the periphery [57, 58]. Evidence suggests both peripheral maturation of class-switched B cells and local maturation within the CSF environment [59, 60]. This indicates that the CSF may serve as a niche for pathogenic T-B cell interactions, further amplifying CNS inflammation. The pivotal role of B cells in MS is underscored by the clinical success of *B-cell-depleting therapies*, which significantly reduce disease activity [61]. Extending single-cell transcriptomic analyses to MS patients undergoing B-cell-depleting therapies or in advanced disease stages could provide deeper insights into the mechanisms of T-B cell crosstalk and immune regulation within the CNS.

The evolving understanding of immune cell composition in CSF highlights the complex interactions between *T cells*, *B cells*, and antigen-presenting cells in MS pathogenesis. The CSF not only serves as a conduit for immune surveillance but also provides a unique environment where immune cells interact, proliferate, and differentiate. The presence of B cell clones, likely resulting from both peripheral influx and local maturation, aligns with the concept of *intrathecal inflammation* in MS. Moreover, the increased abundance of cytotoxic CD4+ T cells and Tregs underscores their potential contributions to both disease exacerbation and immune regulation, respectively. Understanding how immune cells, particularly *CD4+ T cells*, *Tregs*, and *B cells*, interact within the CSF microenvironment will offer critical insights into MS pathology.

4. Meningeal immunity in health and MS

The meninges are highly vascularized tissues composed of three protective layers: the outer dura mater, the middle arachnoid mater, and the inner pia mater [62]. The dura mater, which is fibrous and robust, contains large arteries, veins, and a lymphatic network that allows constituents and cells from the CSF to drain into the lymphatic system [63, 64]. Importantly, paravascular glymphatic fluid flow and meningeal lymphatic drainage of CSF undergo dynamic changes throughout life, playing vital roles in fluid clearance, immune surveillance, and CNS homeostasis [65, 66] (**Figure 3**).

Meningeal immunity refers to the complex integration of immune surveillance and defense mechanisms within the meningeal space, encompassing glymphatic drainage, lymphatic vessels, immune cells, and cytokines [67, 68]. Despite not being directly exposed to the external environment, the meninges act as a gatekeeper by preventing pathogens from infiltrating the CNS. Constant CSF sampling enables immune cells in the meninges to monitor brain homeostasis, detect pathological signals, and trigger appropriate immune responses [64]. Indeed, the meninges are immunologically active hubs, harboring a diverse repertoire of immune cells in both healthy and diseased states. These include T lymphocytes, B lymphocytes, neutrophils, dendritic cells (DCs), macrophages, and mast cells [69–72]. CSF plays a pivotal role in meningeal immunity, as it can access skull bone marrow niches through dura-skull channels, establishing a feedback loop that recruits various immune cells to the meningeal space under both physiological and pathological conditions [4] (**Figure 3**).

Most meningeal immune cells reside in the dura mater, including, dendritic cells, mast cells meningeal macrophages, B cells and T cells. It has been shown that the

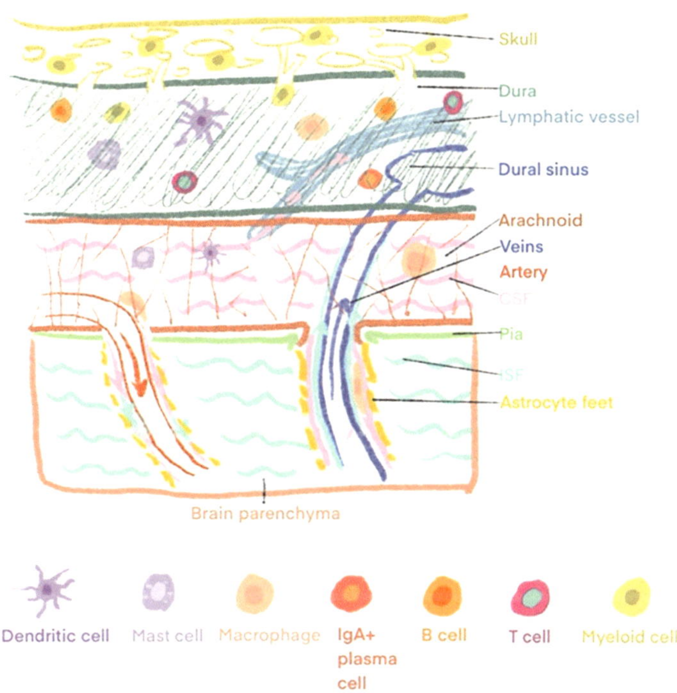

Figure 3.
Meningeal immunity and its cellular compositions. The meninges, composed of the dura, arachnoid, and pia mater, are vascularized tissues that protect the CNS. The dura mater supports lymphatic drainage, facilitating CSF clearance and immune surveillance by lymphatic vessels and the dural sinus. Glymphatic systems dynamically regulate fluid flow and CNS homeostasis. The meninges also host immune cells, including T and B lymphocytes, macrophages, and dendritic cells, enabling immune responses via CSF sampling and dura-skull channels. Myeloid cells migrate to the meninges via vascular channels from bone marrow. DCs and monocytes enrich the dura, while macrophages near meningeal and pial vessels ensure immune surveillance and protection.

migration of myeloid cells into the meninges occurs through specialized vascular channels that connect the meninges to vertebral and calvarial bone marrow [63, 73]. DCs and monocytes are enriched in the dura mater under steady-state conditions [71]. Meningeal macrophages are strategically positioned adjacent to meningeal vessels, while perivascular macrophages line the pial vessels, collectively providing immune surveillance and protection along these critical barrier structures [74, 75]. Notably, the dura also serves as a unique niche for B cell development, housing significant populations of B-lineage progenitors at the pro-B cell stage [76]. Meningeal mature B cells are predominantly naive, and surprisingly, in unchallenged meninges, most perisinus plasma cells were found to be IgA-positive, which contributes to an immunological barrier at this interface, protecting against the spread of pathogens into the CNS [77]. A recent study extended this paradigm, identifying gut-derived IL10-producing IgA^+ plasma cells within the brain and spinal cord during inflammation in a mouse model of multiple sclerosis [78]. Furthermore, scRNA-seq has identified critical chemokine signaling pathways within the meningeal space, such as CCL2/CCL12/CCL8-CCR2 (monocytes), CCL6-CCR1 (neutrophils), and CXCL12-CXCR4 (B cells), emphasizing their role in immune cell recruitment and homeostasis. T cells are largely absent from the CNS parenchyma under steady-state conditions but are abundant in the dura mater. In contrast, they are rarely observed in the choroid plexus [79, 80]. Interestingly, in mice, distinct T cell populations occupy the meninges during different stages of life, with specific functional roles; for example, γδ T cells accumulate in the dura mater during perinatal stages, and αβ T cells (CD4+ and CD8+) accumulate in the meninges after weaning [79].

Meningeal immunity plays a pivotal role in neuroinflammatory diseases such as MS. In MS, early pathological events include BBB leakage and infiltration of CD8+ T cells into the CNS parenchyma, CSF, and meningeal spaces [81, 82]. These infiltrating T cells are predominantly activated in the meninges before migrating into the CNS parenchyma, as demonstrated in experimental autoimmune encephalomyelitis (EAE), a widely used animal model of MS [83]. In both MS patients and EAE models, ectopic lymphoid follicles form within the meninges, and these organized structures consist of immune cell aggregates that provide a favorable environment for T cell reactivation, correlating with disease severity and inflammation [84]. Additionally, adoptive transfer experiments in EAE have demonstrated that T cells first appear in the dura and leptomeninges (the arachnoid and pia mater are sometimes together called the leptomeninges) before the onset of clinical symptoms [85]. This finding underscores the meninges as critical early sites of immune activation during autoimmune inflammation, where T cells are primed and contribute to the progression of CNS pathology [86]. Chronic EAE models further confirmed that T cell infiltration, activation levels, and antigen presentation are more prominent in the leptomeninges than in the dura [87]. In studies of MS patients, meningeal accumulations of *T cells* and *B cells*—but not myeloid cells—were spatially associated with *subpial cortical lesions* [88]. Greater immune cell accumulation correlated with larger lesion areas and more extensive white matter (WM) damage, particularly in active and mixed active/inactive lesions in progressive MS [88]. These findings underscore the role of meningeal lymphocytes in driving subpial cortical injury and their potential link to subcortical white matter.

In summary, in diseases like multiple sclerosis, meningeal immunity is a key player in immune activation, where T and B cells accumulate within the meningeal compartments and drive CNS pathology. While considerable progress has been made in understanding T cell dynamics, the role of B cell-T cell interactions within the meninges remains underexplored. Given the critical role of B cells in MS pathogenesis, as highlighted by the success of B cell-depleting therapies, further investigation into these interactions could provide valuable insights into disease mechanisms and therapeutic strategies in MS.

5. Skull bone marrow in health and MS

The skull bone marrow plays a unique and critical role in the immune dynamics of the CNS. Unlike long bones, which develop via endochondral ossification and sustain load-bearing mechanical stress, the skull develops through intramembranous ossification, giving it distinct structural, functional, and immunological characteristics [89]. This difference enables the skull bone marrow to serve as a specialized immune reservoir with unique responses tailored to the CNS [90–92]. Notably, the skull bone marrow undergoes continuous vascular growth and expansion throughout life, which supports hematopoietic stem cell (HSC) function and ensures finely tuned immune responses that directly influence CNS homeostasis and pathology [93]. Recent advances have revealed direct anatomical and functional connections between the skull bone marrow and CNS, transforming our understanding of neuroimmune interactions (**Figure 4**).

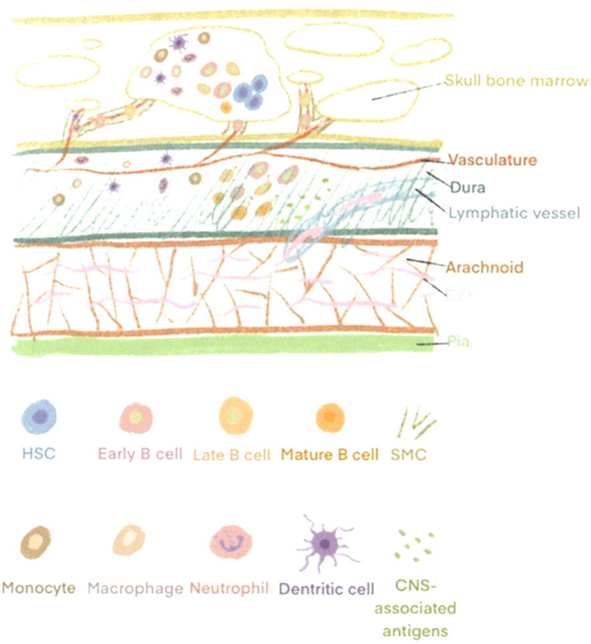

Figure 4.
Skull bone marrow in CNS immunity. The skull bone marrow supports hematopoietic stem cell (HSC) function and CNS immunity through vascular channels called skull-meningeal connections (SMCs). These channels link the dura to bone marrow, enabling immune cell migration for surveillance. Since the meninges are in contact with CSF when drainage to lymphatic vessels, molecules from the CNS can reach B cells in the skull bone marrow, exposing them to CNS-related antigens. Naïve B cell in dura can be educated by this exposure to reduce autoreactive B cells. Moreover, skull bone marrow can facilitate the meningeal B cells development and differentiation but rather from circulating blood.

The dura mater, the outermost meningeal layer, is connected to the skull bone marrow through specialized skull-meningeal connections (SMCs). These vascular channels allow immune cells to traffic from the skull bone marrow to the meninges, creating a direct pathway for immune surveillance and response [2, 18, 20]. The channels, originating at the inner cortex of the skull and extending into the marrow cavities, link the dural vasculature to the sinusoidal vasculature of the bone marrow [2, 4]. In mice, these channels are distributed across the frontal, parietal, and occipital bones, measuring 20–25 μm in width [2, 4, 17, 18, 20, 94]. In humans, micro-CT imaging has revealed similar structures, with channels four- to five-fold larger in diameter than those in mice, allowing greater immune cell migration capacity. These connections enable rapid immune responses to perturbations in the CNS, highlighting the skull bone marrow's role as a dynamic immune reservoir (**Figure 4**).

The skull and vertebral bone marrow supply immune cells, such as monocytes, neutrophils, macrophages, and dendritic cells, to the meninges and CNS [2, 4, 18, 20]. These cells, delivered via direct dura-bone marrow channels, are integral to immune surveillance, inflammation, and tissue repair under both normal and pathological conditions. For example, during neuroinflammation, immune cells originating from the skull bone marrow exhibit distinct phenotypes compared to blood-derived counterparts, influencing disease progression and severity. In a mouse model of MS, autoreactive T cells have been observed to migrate to the bone marrow, where they amplify myelopoiesis through the CCL5-CCR5 axis. This process increases the proliferation of CCR5+ myeloid-biased hematopoietic stem and progenitor cells [95]; subsequently, elevated myeloid cell exacerbates CNS inflammation, contributing to the progression of neuroinflammatory pathology in MS. Consistent with this enhanced marrow activation, TSPO-PET imaging of patients with primary progressive and relapsing-remitting MS shows significant enhancement in the skull marrow [19]. This finding underscores the importance of the skull bone marrow in shaping the immune landscape of the CNS.

Parabiosis experiments and single-cell RNA sequencing (scRNA-seq) have revealed that meningeal immune cells, particularly B cells, comprise approximately 30% of CD45+ cells in mouse meninges, including both immature and mature B cells within the dural tissue. Meningeal B cells have been further characterized into three developmental subsets: early B cells (CD19 + B220loCD43hi), late B cells (CD19 + B220loCD43lo), and mature B cells (CD19 + B220hiCD43−). Comparative analyses of meningeal B cells with B cells from the bone marrow (BM), blood, and spleen demonstrated a similar distribution of these subsets in the meninges and BM. Early B cells in both compartments were identified as IgM − CD93+, mature B cells as IgM + CD93−, and late B cells exhibited an intermediate phenotype. In contrast, B cells in the blood and spleen predominantly displayed a mature phenotype [4, 96].

These findings suggest that meningeal B cells do not primarily originate from circulating blood but rather develop within the skull bone marrow. Meningeal B cells span various developmental stages, from pro-B cells to mature B lymphocytes, and exhibit characteristics distinct from peripheral blood B cells. This indicates that the skull bone marrow serves as a specialized niche for B cell development and differentiation, playing a critical role in CNS immune regulation [4, 96]. Additionally, the dura mater harbors a significant population of these B cells, further emphasizing the central role of skull bone marrow in maintaining CNS immunity.

Beyond acting as a myeloid reservoir, the skull bone marrow is also central to maintaining CNS tolerance. For instance, it is a site for lymphopoiesis, supplying both immature and mature B cells to the underlying dural tissue. Because the meninges have access to CSF, molecules from the CNS can interact with B cells in the skull bone marrow, exposing them to CNS-associated antigens [17, 49, 50, 97] such as myelin oligodendrocyte glycoprotein (MOG) (**Figure 4**). This exposure facilitates the negative selection of autoreactive B cells, thereby reducing autoimmune reactions. However, disruptions in this process could lead to the persistence of autoreactive lymphocytes, exacerbating autoimmune diseases like MS.

In conclusion, the skull bone marrow represents a critical component of CNS immune regulation, contributing to both surveillance and inflammation at the CNS borders. Its unique anatomical and functional characteristics highlight its importance in maintaining CNS homeostasis and underscore its potential as a therapeutic target in neuroinflammatory diseases. Understanding the interplay between skull bone marrow and the CNS will pave the way for innovative strategies to address conditions like MS and other neuroimmune disorders.

6. Unanswered questions

Although significant progress has been made in understanding the role of skull bone marrow in CNS immunity, many questions remain unanswered:

- How does the skull-derived immune response influence T cell-B cell interactions within the CNS, particularly in MS patients?
- Are there specific signaling pathways or molecular markers that distinguish skull-derived immune responses from peripheral immune responses?
- In what ways might dysregulated skull immunity exacerbate neuroinflammatory conditions like MS?
- What role do environmental or genetic factors play in influencing skull immunity and its interactions with the CNS?
- How does immune cell composition within the skull bone marrow change during neuroinflammation or disease progression in MS?
- Are there differences in skull immunity across different stages of MS (e.g., relapsing-remitting vs. progressive MS)?
- Can skull immunity be selectively targeted for therapeutic interventions without affecting systemic immunity?

7. Conclusions

The paradigm shift from viewing the CNS as an immune-privileged organ to recognizing its intricate connection with the immune system has fundamentally reshaped our understanding of neuroimmune dynamics. The skull bone marrow and its related meningeal immunity, as an immune cell reservoir uniquely adapted to CNS needs, plays a central role in these interactions. Its ability to respond rapidly to CNS perturbations underscores its importance in both homeostasis and pathology. Further studies are needed to uncover the mechanisms driving skull bone marrow-mediated immune responses, such as B-T cell interaction, particularly in diseases like MS, where these processes may offer novel therapeutic targets.

Conflict of interest

The authors declare no conflict of interest.

Author details

Yawei Liu, Xinchen Nie and Henrik Hasseldam*
Biotech Research and Innovation Centre (BRIC), Faculty of Health and Medical Sciences, University of Copenhagen, Copenhagen N, Denmark

*Address all correspondence to: henrik.hasseldam@bric.ku.dk

References

[1] Trobisch T, Kutza M, Ludwig N, Wischnewski S, Zulji A, Lerma-Martin C, et al. Cell-cell interaction networks and meningeal inflammation in progressive multiple sclerosis. Multiple Sclerosis Journal. 2024;**30**(3):485

[2] Cugurra A, Mamuladze T, Rustenhoven J, Dykstra T, Beroshvili G, Greenberg ZJ, et al. Skull and vertebral bone marrow are myeloid cell reservoirs for the meninges and CNS parenchyma. Science. 2021;**373**(6553):409

[3] Mazzitelli JA, Pulous FE, Smyth LCD, Kaya Z, Rustenhoven J, Moskowitz MA, et al. Skull bone marrow channels as immune gateways to the central nervous system. Nature Neuroscience. 2023;**26**(12):2052-2062

[4] Brioschi S, Wang WL, Peng V, Wang M, Shchukina I, Greenberg ZJ, et al. Heterogeneity of meningeal B cells reveals a lymphopoietic niche at the CNS borders. Science. 2021;**373**(6553):408

[5] Louveau A. Meningeal immunity, drainage, and tertiary lymphoid structure formation. Methods in Molecular Biology. 2018;**1845**:31-45

[6] Rua R, Lee J, Silva A, Dragan M, Johnson K, McGavern DB. Meningeal inflammation drives long-term engraftment by monocytes that impair CNS immunity. Journal of Immunology. 2018;**200**(1_Supplement):168.4

[7] Hu XT, Deng QP, Ma L, Li QQ, Chen YD, Liao YH, et al. Meningeal lymphatic vessels regulate brain tumor drainage and immunity. Cell Research. 2020;**30**(3):229-243

[8] Rubin M, Pagani E, Meani A, Preziosa P, Storelli L, Margoni M, et al. Different CSF-in gradients of damage occur in the thalamus, caudate nucleus and cortex in multiple sclerosis: A 3T magnetization transfer ratio and R2*study. Multiple Sclerosis Journal. 2023;**29**:247-248

[9] Verdiani A, Picozza M, Mazziotti V, Turano E, Virla F, Marastoni D, et al. Functional and phenotypic flow cytometry analysis of immune cells in CSF and whole blood of patients with multiple sclerosis. Multiple Sclerosis Journal. 2023;**29**:814

[10] Dekeyser C, Hautekeete M, Cambron M, Van Pesch V, Patti F, Kuhle J, et al. Routine CSF parameters as predictors of disease course in multiple sclerosis: An MSBase cohort study. Journal of Neurology, Neurosurgery and Psychiatry. 2024;**95**(11):1021-1031

[11] Haase S, Linker RA. Inflammation in multiple sclerosis. Therapeutic Advances in Neurological Disorders. 2021;**14**:17562864211007687

[12] Cacciaguerra L, Curatoli C, Vizzino C, Valsasina P, Filippi M, Rocca MA. Functional correlates of cognitive abilities vary with age in pediatric multiple sclerosis. Multiple Sclerosis and Related Disorders. 2024;**82**:105404

[13] Opsommer E, Ribeiro C, Carrard S, Hilfiker R, Mbarga J. Exploring the integration and patient engagement of balance home exercises in the daily management of multiple sclerosis: A comprehensive qualitative analysis. Disability and Rehabilitation. 2024:1-9

[14] Lafta MS, Sokolov AV, Landtblom AM, Ericson H, Schioeth HB, Abu Hamdeh S. Exploring biomarkers in

trigeminal neuralgia patients operated with microvascular decompression: A comparison with multiple sclerosis patients and non-neurological controls. European Journal of Pain. 2024;**28**(6):929-942

[15] Jovanovic A, Pekmezovic T, Mesaros S, Novakovic I, Peterlin B, Veselinovic N, et al. Exclusive breastfeeding may be a protective factor in individuals with familial multiple sclerosis. A population registry-based case-control study. Multiple Sclerosis and Related Disorders. 2024;**82**:105392

[16] Vudumula U, Patidar M, Gudala K, Karpf E, Adlard N. Evaluating the impact of early vs delayed ofatumumab initiation and estimating the long-term outcomes of ofatumumab vs teriflunomide in relapsing multiple sclerosis patients in Spain. Journal of Medical Economics. 2023;**26**(1):11-18

[17] Mazzitelli JA, Smyth LCD, Cross KA, Dykstra T, Sun J, Du SL, et al. Cerebrospinal fluid regulates skull bone marrow niches via direct access through dural channels. Nature Neuroscience. 2022;**25**(5):555

[18] Herisson F, Frodermann V, Courties G, Rohde D, Sun Y, Vandoorne K, et al. Direct vascular channels connect skull bone marrow and the brain surface enabling myeloid cell migration. Nature Neuroscience. 2018;**21**(9):1209-1217

[19] Kolabas ZI, Kuemmerle LB, Perneczky R, Förstera B, Ulukaya S, Ali M, et al. Distinct molecular profiles of skull bone marrow in health and neurological disorders. Cell. 2023;**186**(17):3706-3725.e29

[20] Cai RY, Pan CC, Ghasemigharagoz A, Todorov MI, Förstera B, Zhao S, et al. Panoptic imaging of transparent mice reveals whole-body neuronal projections and skull-meninges connections. Nature Neuroscience. 2019;**22**(2):317

[21] Louyeau A, Harris TH, Kipnis J. Revisiting the mechanisms of CNS immune privilege. Trends in Immunology. 2015;**36**(10):569-577

[22] Medawar PB. Immunity to homologous grafted skin. 3. The fate of skin homografts transplanted to the brain, to subcutaneous tissue, and to the anterior chamber of the eye. British Journal of Experimental Pathology. 1948;**29**(1):58

[23] Ransohoff RM, Kivisäkk P, Kidd G. Three or more routes for leukocyte migration into the central nervous system. Nature Reviews. Immunology. 2003;**3**(7):569-581

[24] Engelhardt B, Ransohoff RM. Capture, crawl, cross: The T cell code to breach the blood-brain barriers. Trends in Immunology. 2012;**33**(12):579-589

[25] Takeshita Y, Ransohoff RM. Inflammatory cell trafficking across the blood-brain barrier: Chemokine regulation and in vitro models. Immunological Reviews. 2012;**248**:228-239

[26] Bentivoglio M, Kristensson K. Tryps and trips: Cell trafficking across the 100-year-old blood-brain barrier. Trends in Neurosciences. 2014;**37**(6):325-333

[27] Weller RO, Djuanda E, Yow HY, Carare RO. Lymphatic drainage of the brain and the pathophysiology of neurological disease. Acta Neuropathologica. 2009;**117**(1):1-14

[28] Laman JD, Weller RO. Drainage of cells and soluble antigen from the CNS to regional lymph nodes. Journal of Neuroimmune Pharmacology. 2013;**8**(4):840-856

[29] Weller RO, Galea I, Carare RO, Minagar A. Pathophysiology of the lymphatic drainage of the central nervous system: Implications for pathogenesis and therapy of multiple sclerosis. Pathophysiology. 2010;**17**(4):295-306

[30] Laman JD, Weller RO. Editorial: Route by which monocytes leave the brain is revealed. Journal of Leukocyte Biology. 2012;**92**(1):6-9

[31] Alghanimy A, Work LM, Holmes WM. The glymphatic system and multiple sclerosis: An evolving connection. Multiple Sclerosis and Related Disorders. 2024;**83**:105456

[32] Iliff JJ, Wang MH, Liao YH, Plogg BA, Peng WG, Gundersen GA, et al. A Paravascular pathway facilitates CSF flow through the brain parenchyma and the clearance of interstitial solutes, including amyloid β. Science Translational Medicine. 2012;**4**(147):147ra111

[33] Iliff J, Simon M. CrossTalk proposal: The glymphatic system supports convective exchange of cerebrospinal fluid and brain interstitial fluid that is mediated by perivascular aquaporin-4. Journal of Physiology (London). 2019;**597**(17):4417-4419

[34] Fournier AP, Gauberti M, Quenault A, Vivien D, Macrez R, Docagne F. Reduced spinal cord parenchymal cerebrospinal fluid circulation in experimental autoimmune encephalomyelitis. Journal of Cerebral Blood Flow & Metabolism. 2019;**39**(7):1258-1265

[35] Schubert JJ, Veronese M, Marchitelli L, Bodini B, Tonietto M, Stankoff B, et al. Dynamic C-PiB PET shows cerebrospinal fluid flow alterations in Alzheimer disease and multiple sclerosis. Journal of Nuclear Medicine. 2019;**60**(10):1452-1460

[36] Carotenuto A, Cacciaguerra L, Pagani E, Preziosa P, Filippi M, Rocca MA. Glymphatic system impairment in multiple sclerosis: Relation with brain damage and disability. Brain. 2022;**145**(8):2785-2795

[37] Cai XZ, Qiao J, Kulkarni P, Harding IC, Ebong E, Ferris CF. Imaging the effect of the circadian light-dark cycle on the glymphatic system in awake rats. Proceedings of the National Academy of Sciences of the United States of America. 2020;**117**(1):668-676

[38] Buratti L, Iacobucci DE, Viticchi G, Falsetti L, Lattanzi S, Pulcini A, et al. Sleep quality can influence the outcome of patients with multiple sclerosis. Sleep Medicine. 2019;**58**:56-60

[39] Mestre H, Hablitz LM, Xavier ALR, Feng WX, Zou WY, Pu TL, et al. Aquaporin-4-dependent glymphatic solute transport in the rodent brain. eLife. 2018;**7**

[40] Granberg T, Moridi T, Brand JS, Neumann S, Hlavica M, Piehl F, et al. Enlarged perivascular spaces in multiple sclerosis on magnetic resonance imaging: A systematic review and meta-analysis. Journal of Neurology. 2020;**267**(11):3199-3212

[41] Gabr RE, Lincoln JA, Hasan KM, Kramer LA. Functional assessment of the dural lymphatic vessels using dynamic contrast MRI in multiple sclerosis. Brain and Behavior: A Cognitive Neuroscience Perspective. 2023;**13**(7):e3042

[42] Tuulasvaara A, Kurdo G, Martola J, Laakso SM. Cervical lymph node diameter reflects disease progression in multiple sclerosis. Multiple Sclerosis and Related Disorders. 2024;**84**

[43] Wolvers DAW, Coenen-de Roo CJJ, Mebius RE, van der Cammen MJF,

Tirion F, Miltenburg AMM, et al. Intranasally induced immunological tolerance is determined by characteristics of the draining lymph nodes: Studies with OVA and human cartilage gp-39. Journal of Immunology. 1999;**162**(4):1994-1998

[44] Phillips MJ, Needham M, Weller RO. Role of cervical lymph nodes in autoimmune encephalomyelitis in the Lewis rat. The Journal of Pathology. 1997;**182**(4):457-464

[45] Furtado GC, Marcondes MCG, Latkowski JA, Tsai J, Wensky A, Lafaille JJ. Swift entry of myelin-specific T lymphocytes into the central nervous system in spontaneous autoimmune encephalomyelitis. Journal of Immunology. 2008;**181**(7):4648-4655

[46] de Vos AF, van Meurs M, Brok HP, Boven LA, Hintzen RQ, van der Valk P, et al. Transfer of central nervous system autoantigens and presentation in secondary lymphoid organs. Journal of Immunology. 2002;**169**(10):5415-5423

[47] van Zwam M, Huizinga R, Melief MJ, Wierenga-Wolf A, van Meurs M, Voerman JS, et al. Brain antigens in functionally distinct antigen-presenting cell populations in cervical lymph nodes in MS and EAE. Journal of Molecular Medicine. 2009;**87**(3):273-286

[48] Bakoyiannis I. CSF: A key player in brain's immunity. Lab Animal. 2022;**51**(7):186

[49] Ringstad G, Eide PK. Cerebrospinal fluid tracer efflux to parasagittal dura in humans. Nature. Communications. 2020;**11**(1):354

[50] Rustenhoven J, Drieu A, Mamuladze T, de Lima KA, Dykstra T, Wall M, et al. Functional characterization of the dural sinuses as a neuroimmune interface. Cell. 2021;**184**(4):1000

[51] Piehl N, van Olst L, Ramakrishnan A, Teregulova V, Simonton B, Zhang ZY, et al. Cerebrospinal fluid immune dysregulation during healthy brain aging and cognitive impairment. Cell. 2022;**185**(26):5028

[52] Theisen DJ, Davidson JT, Briseño CG, Gargaro M, Lauron EJ, Wang QL, et al. WDFY4 is required for cross-presentation in response to viral and tumor antigens. Science. 2018;**362**(6415):694

[53] Schafflick D, Xu CLA, Hartlehnert M, Cole M, Schulte-Mecklenbeck A, Lautwein T, et al. Integrated single cell analysis of blood and cerebrospinal fluid leukocytes in multiple sclerosis. Nature Communications. 2020;**11**(1):247

[54] Patil VS, Madrigal A, Schmiedel BJ, Clarke J, O'Rourke P, de Silva AD, et al. Precursors of human CD4 cytotoxic T lymphocytes identified by single-cell transcriptome analysis. Science Immunology. 2018;**3**(19):eaan8664

[55] Enose-Akahata Y, Azodi S, Smith B, Billioux B, Vellucci A, Ngouth N, et al. Immunophenotypic characterization of CSF B cells in virus-associated neuroinflammatory diseases. Journal of Neurovirology. 2018;**24**:S26-S

[56] Corcione A, Casazza S, Ferretti E, Giunti D, Zappia E, Pistorio A, et al. Recapitulation of B cell differentiation in the central nervous system of patients with multiple sclerosis. Proceedings of the National Academy of Sciences of the United States of America. 2004;**101**(30):11064-11069

[57] Von Budingen H, Kuo T, Sirota M, van Belle C, Apeltsin L, Glanville J, et al.

B cell exchange across the blood-brain barrier in multiple sclerosis. Neurology. 2013;**80**(7_supplement):S11.003

[58] Eggers EL, Michel BA, Wu H, Wang SZ, Bevan CJ, Abounasr A, et al. Clonal relationships of CSF B cells in treatment-naive multiple sclerosis patients. JCI Insight. 2017;**2**(22):e92724

[59] Palanichamy A, Apeltsin L, Kuo TC, Sirota M, Wang SZ, Pitts SJ, et al. Immunoglobulin class-switched B cells form an active immune axis between CNS and periphery in multiple sclerosis. Science Translational Medicine. 2014;**6**(248):248ra106

[60] Stern JNH, Yaari G, Vander Heiden JA, Church G, Donahue WF, Hintzen RQ, et al. B cells populating the multiple sclerosis brain mature in the draining cervical lymph nodes. Science Translational Medicine. 2014;**6**(248):248ra107

[61] Hauser SL, Bar-Or A, Comi G, Giovannoni G, Hartung HP, Hemmer B, et al. Ocrelizumab versus interferon Beta-1a in relapsing multiple sclerosis. The New England Journal of Medicine. 2017;**376**(3):221-234

[62] Magliozzi R, Howell OW, Calabrese M, Reynolds R. Meningeal inflammation as a driver of cortical grey matter pathology and clinical progression in multiple sclerosis. Nature Reviews. Neurology. 2023;**19**(8):461-476

[63] Louveau A, Smirnov I, Keyes TJ, Eccles JD, Rouhani SJ, Peske JD, et al. Structural and functional features of central nervous system lymphatic vessels. Nature. 2015;**523**(7560):337

[64] de Lima KA, Rustenhoven J, Kipnis J. Meningeal immunity and its function in maintenance of the central nervous system in health and disease. Annual Review of Immunology. 2020;**38**:597-620

[65] Kress BT, Iliff JJ, Xia MS, Wang MH, Wei HLS, Zeppenfeld D, et al. Impairment of paravascular clearance pathways in the aging brain. Annals of Neurology. 2014;**76**(6):845-861

[66] Da Mesquita S, Louveau A, Vaccari A, Smirnov I, Cornelison RC, Kingsmore KM, et al. Functional aspects of meningeal lymphatics in ageing and Alzheimer's disease. Nature. 2018;**560**(7717):185

[67] Ma TY, Wang FS, Xu SJ, Huang JH. Meningeal immunity: Structure, function and a potential therapeutic target of neurodegenerative diseases. Brain, Behavior, and Immunity. 2021;**93**:264-276

[68] de Lima KA, Rustenhoven J, Da Mesquita S, Wall M, Salvador A, Smirnov I, et al. Meningeal γδ T cells regulate anxiety-like behavior via IL-17a signaling in neurons. Biological Psychiatry. 2021;**89**(9):S65-S

[69] Filiano AJ, Gadani SP, Kipnis J. How and why do T cells and their derived cytokines affect the injured and healthy brain? Nature Reviews. Neuroscience. 2017;**18**(6):375-384

[70] Tanabe S, Yamashita T. B-1a lymphocytes promote oligodendrogenesis during brain development. Nature Neuroscience. 2018;**21**(4):506

[71] Van Hove H, Martens L, Scheyltjens I, De Vlaminck K, Antunes ARP, De Prijck S, et al. A single-cell atlas of mouse brain macrophages reveals unique transcriptional identities shaped by ontogeny and tissue environment. Nature Neuroscience. 2019;**22**(6):1021-1035

[72] Ding XB, Wang XX, Xia DH, Liu H, Tian HY, Fu Y, et al. Impaired meningeal lymphatic drainage in patients with

idiopathic Parkinson's disease. Nature Medicine. 2021;**27**(3):411

[73] Goldmann T, Wieghofer P, Jordao MJC, Prutek F, Hagemeyer N, Frenzel K, et al. Origin, fate and dynamics of macrophages at central nervous system interfaces. Nature Immunology. 2016;**17**(7):797

[74] Polfliet MMJ, Zwijnenburg PJG, van Furth AM, van der Poll T, Döpp EA, de Lavalette CR, et al. Meningeal and perivascular macrophages of the central nervous system play a protective role during bacterial meningitis. Journal of Immunology. 2001;**167**(8):4644-4650

[75] Herz J, Filiano AJ, Wiltbank AT, Yogev N, Kipnis J. Myeloid cells in the central nervous system. Immunity. 2017;**46**(6):943-956

[76] Schafflick D, Wolbert J, Heming M, Thomas C, Hartlehnert M, Börsch AL, et al. Single-cell profiling of CNS border compartment leukocytes reveals that B cells and their progenitors reside in non-diseased meninges. Nature Neuroscience. 2021;**24**(9):1225-1234

[77] Fitzpatrick Z, Frazer G, Ferro A, Clare S, Bouladoux N, Ferdinand J, et al. Gut-educated IgA plasma cells defend the meningeal venous sinuses. Nature. 2020;**587**(7834):472

[78] Rojas OL, Pröbstel AK, Porfilio EA, Wang AA, Charabati M, Sun T, et al. Recirculating intestinal IgA-producing cells regulate neuroinflammation via IL-10. Cell. 2019;**176**:610. 2019; 177(2):492-3

[79] Ribeiro M, Brigas HC, Temido-Ferreira M, Pousinha PA, Regen T, Santa C, et al. Meningeal γδ T cell-derived IL-17 controls synaptic plasticity and short-term memory. Science Immunology. 2019;**4**(40):eaay5199

[80] de Lima KA, Rustenhoven J, Da Mesquita S, Wall M, Salvador AF, Smirnov I, et al. Meningeal γδ T cells regulate anxiety-like behavior via IL-17a signaling in neurons. Nature Immunology. 2020;**21**(11):1421

[81] Giunti D, Borsellino G, Benelli R, Marchese M, Capello E, Valle MT, et al. Phenotypic and functional analysis of T cells homing into the CSF of subjects with inflammatory diseases of the CNS. Journal of Leukocyte Biology. 2003;**73**(5):584-590

[82] Alvermann S, Hennig C, Stüve O, Wiendl H, Stangel M. Immunophenotyping of cerebrospinal fluid cells in multiple sclerosis in search of biomarkers. JAMA Neurology. 2014;**71**(7):905-912

[83] Schläger C, Körner H, Krueger M, Vidoli S, Haberl M, Mielke D, et al. Effector T-cell trafficking between the leptomeninges and the cerebrospinal fluid. Nature. 2016;**530**(7590):349

[84] Russi AE, Brown MA. The meninges: New therapeutic targets for multiple sclerosis. Translational Research. 2015;**165**(2):255-269

[85] Walker-Caulfield ME, Hatfield JK, Brown MA. Dynamic changes in meningeal inflammation correspond to clinical exacerbations in a murine model of relapsing-remitting multiple sclerosis. Journal of Neuroimmunology. 2015;**278**:112-122

[86] Kwong B, Rua R, Gao YY, Flickinger J, Wang Y, Kruhlak MJ, et al. T-bet-dependent NKp46^{+} innate lymphoid cells regulate the onset of T17-induced neuroinflammation. Nature Immunology. 2017;**18**:1117. 2018; 19(8):898

[87] Merlini A, Haberl M, Strauss J, Hildebrand L, Genc N, Franz J,

et al. Distinct roles of the meningeal layers in CNS autoimmunity. Nature Neuroscience. 2022;**25**(7):887

[88] Ahmed SM, Fransen NL, Touil H, Michailidou I, Huitinga I, Gommerman JL, et al. Accumulation of meningeal lymphocytes correlates with white matter lesion activity in progressive multiple sclerosis. JCI Insight. 2022;**7**(5):e151683

[89] Yuan GX, Lin XX, Liu Y, Greenblatt MB, Xu R. Skeletal stem cells in bone development, homeostasis, and disease. Protein & Cell. 2024;**15**(8):559-574

[90] Comazzetto S, Shen B, Morrison SJ. Niches that regulate stem cells and hematopoiesis in adult bone marrow. Developmental Cell. 2021;**56**(13):1848-1860

[91] van den Bos T, Speijer D, Bank RA, Brömme D, Everts V. Differences in matrix composition between calvaria and long bone in mice suggest differences in biomechanical properties and resorption special emphasis on collagen. Bone. 2008;**43**(3):459-468

[92] Sivaraj KK, Adams RH. Blood vessel formation and function in bone. Development. 2016;**143**(15):2706-2715

[93] Koh BI, Mohanakrishnan V, Jeong HW, Park H, Kruse K, Choi YJ, et al. Adult skull bone marrow is an expanding and resilient haematopoietic reservoir. Nature. Dec 2024;**636**(8041):172-181

[94] Yao H, Price TT, Cantelli G, Ngo B, Warner MJ, Olivere L, et al. Leukaemia hijacks a neural mechanism to invade the central nervous system. Nature. 2018;**560**(7716):55

[95] Shi KB, Li HD, Chang T, He WY, Kong Y, Qi CY, et al. Bone marrow hematopoiesis drives multiple sclerosis progression. Cell. 2022;**185**(13):2234

[96] Wang Y, Chen DY, Xu D, Huang C, Xing RX, He DY, et al. Early developing B cells undergo negative selection by central nervous system-specific antigens in the meninges. Immunity. 2021;**54**(12):2784

[97] Pulous FE, Cruz-Hernández JC, Yang CB, Kaya Z, Paccalet A, Wojtkiewicz G, et al. Cerebrospinal fluid can exit into the skull bone marrow and instruct cranial hematopoiesis in mice with bacterial meningitis. Nature Neuroscience. 2022;**25**(5):567

Section 2

Presentation and Diagnosis

Chapter 3

Multi-Omics Profiling of Cerebrospinal Fluid: A Strategy for Unveiling Multiple Sclerosis

Kleiton de Barros Borges, Victória Regina da Silva, Jordana Marina da Silva, Valéria Visani, Maria Helena Menezes Estevam Alves and Danyelly Bruneska Gondim Martins

Abstract

Multiple sclerosis is an inflammatory and chronic disease of the central nervous system. It affects about 3 million people worldwide, primarily young patients, and unfortunately remains without a cure. Cerebrospinal fluid plays a key role in the diagnostic work-up, helping to reduce the chances of misdiagnosis, some of them caused by misinterpretation of neuroimaging results. The revision of the McDonald criteria in 2024 indicates two key parameters that must be evaluated in the cerebrospinal fluid of patients with multiple sclerosis, oligoclonal bands and the kappa index. Indeed, cerebrospinal fluid envelops various structures of the central nervous system and contains traces of proteins, immunoglobulins, and small molecules capable of crossing the blood-brain barrier, making it useful in clinical practice. Therefore, a multi-omics profiling of cerebrospinal fluid can contribute to the development of new diagnostic markers, as well as monitoring the therapeutic failure of disease-modifying drugs. It enables more targeted treatment, better outcomes for the patient, and a lower economic burden for funding organizations. This chapter intends to discuss the potential of different omics approaches and related technologies to identify biomarkers in cerebrospinal fluid.

Keywords: translational science, omics, biomarkers, differential diagnosis, targeted-therapy

1. Introduction

Multiple sclerosis (MS) is an inflammatory disease of the central nervous system (CNS) characterized by elevated degree of heterogeneity regarding clinical manifestations, disease course, radiologic and cerebrospinal fluid (CSF) findings.

IntechOpen

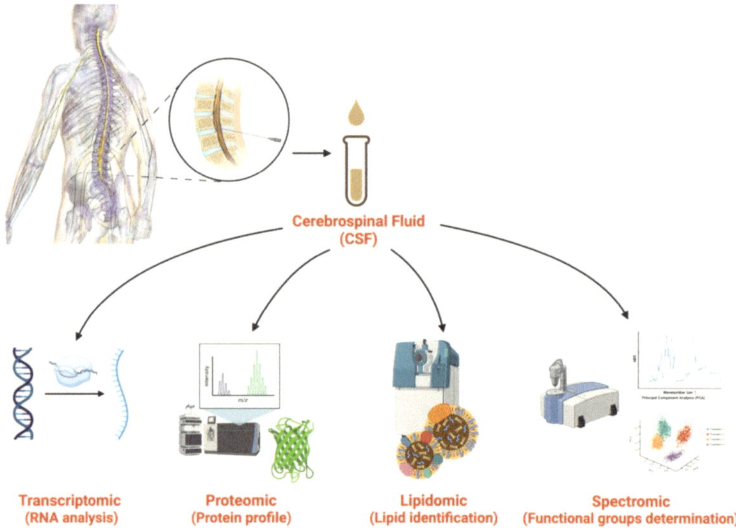

Figure 1.
Scheme cerebrospinal fluid sampling and possible omic-based techniques that can be used for understanding about multiple sclerosis and identifying different biomarkers.

The pathophysiology of MS is multifactorial, and not fully understood. It is believed that genetic and environmental factors, such as Epstein-Barr virus infection, vitamin D deficiency, and smoking habits, contribute to an increased risk of developing this disease [1]. Clinically, patients may show gradual progress of disability, either at disease onset (primary progressive MS—PPMS) or after a relapsing-remitting course (secondary progressive MS—SPMS). There is no specific biomarker for the disease, so the diagnosis relies on clinical evaluation alongside the observation of lesions *via* magnetic resonance imaging (MRI). The diagnostic is supported by other paraclinical methods such as cerebrospinal fluid analysis, which provides essential information for the differential diagnosis. It is important to avoid misdiagnostic conditions that mimic MS, like the presence of intrathecal IgG synthesis [2] that specifically indicates a high probability of conversion to MS after a clinically isolated syndrome (CIS) [3]. Nevertheless, it is still difficult to associate the clinical symptoms to MS at first evaluation, leading to a delay in the efficient treatment. Some doubts can be answered with the use of different molecular study techniques, the multi-omics, which includes the analysis of gene transcription, protein, and lipid expression, that can be associated with spectrophotometry studies and indicate the disease molecular profile (**Figure 1**).

2. Molecular aspects of CSF in multiple sclerosis

The value of CSF analysis for the diagnosis of multiple sclerosis is well-established, once it better reflects the inflammatory environment of the CNS compared to blood analysis [4]. The analysis of CSF also provides greater accuracy in detecting locoregional evidence of inflammation compared to methods like MRI, especially in cases where the disease is not highly active [5]. Moreover, it is important to highlight its potential role in a comprehensive assessment of the disease course, through the evaluation of diagnostic parameters of inflammation (oligoclonal bands and kappa-free light chains) and axonal damage (neurofilament light chain).

2.1 Oligoclonal bands

The search for oligoclonal bands (OCBs) is an important parameter for detecting humoral response in the CNS. OCBs are composed of immunoglobulin clones produced by plasma cells, indicating an antigenic response associated with inflammatory as well as infectious diseases [6]. When restricted to the CSF, within an appropriate clinical context, they support the diagnosis of MS. According to the revised 2017 McDonald criteria, two or more oligoclonal bands restricted to the CSF indicate a high likelihood of conversion to MS and may suggest that the criterion of dissemination in time has been met [7]. The authors of the revised 2017 McDonald criteria emphasize that the methodology used is crucial for improving the accuracy of the test. The preferred methodology is agarose gel electrophoresis with isoelectric focusing and immunoblotting or immunofixation for IgG [2].

From a practical perspective, to determine that OCBs are specific to CSF, it is necessary to collect a serum sample in parallel. Without serum, it is impossible to establish a reliable result. Another important precaution is to avoid blood contamination in the CSF, which can occur in traumatic taps. This can increase the amount of polyclonal IgG derived from blood. In such cases, it is essential to inform the laboratory and interpret the results with caution [8]. The analysis of OCBs should always be performed in an appropriate clinical context, once they may be present in healthy individuals and in non-inflammatory conditions, such as idiopathic intracranial hypertension [9]. Therefore, clinical correlation is mandatory to avoid misdiagnosis, and five possible patterns can be identified in the analysis of oligoclonal bands (**Figure 2**):

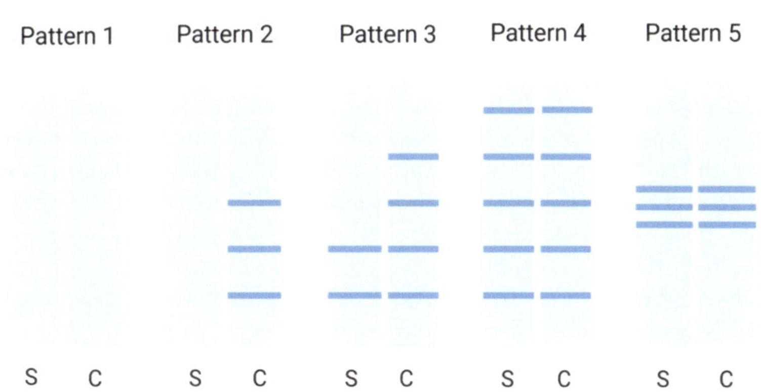

Figure 2.
Schematic representation of oligoclonal band patterns obtained by agarose gel electrophoresis with isoelectric focusing and immunoblotting or immunofixation for IgG. This enables a more detailed analysis instead of merely classifying OCBs as "negative" or "positive." S = serum, C = CSF.

- Pattern 1—Absence of OCBs in both serum and CSF, though a polyclonal IgG distribution may be present

- Pattern 2—OCBs are present in CSF, but absent in serum (indicating intrathecal synthesis, as OCB positivity)
- Pattern 3—OCBs are present in both CSF and serum, but some additional identical OCB only in CSF
- Pattern 4—Identical OCBs are present in CSF and serum ("mirror pattern")
- Pattern 5—Monoclonal bands in CSF and serum (presence of monoclonal gammopathy)

Considering the diagnosis of MS, approximately 90% of patients exhibit the presence of OCBs, and patterns types 2 and 3 are the most common. Therefore, it is mandatory to conduct a thorough investigation for MS mimics when OCBs are absent. Albeit less commonly, OCBs may also be present in other inflammatory conditions such as neuromyelitis optica spectrum disorder (NMOSD) [10] and myelin oligodendrocyte glycoprotein-associated disease (MOGAD) [11].

2.2 Kappa-free light chain

It is known that B cells produce immunoglobulins through the linkage of light and heavy chains. However, they also produce free light chains (FLC), which, in cases of chronic inflammation such as MS, are found in excess and may have diagnostic value [12]. Indeed, the determination of intrathecal synthesis of **κ**-FLC was widely discussed at the latest ECTRIMS conference in 2024 and is expected to be included in the new McDonald criteria as a diagnostic tool. Evidence shows that **κ**-FLC has similar accuracy compared to OCBs, with a sensitivity and specificity of 90%. Moreover, it is easy to perform and can also predict disease activity in MS [13].

2.3 Neurofilament light chain

Neurofilaments are cytoskeletal proteins that can indicate axonal damage. These molecules are not exclusive to patients with MS; once different conditions can cause cellular damage, such as stroke or other neurodegenerative diseases [14] can also increase their levels. Although neurofilaments do not have significant diagnostic value, it seems to play a better role in predicting relapse risk and monitoring the effectiveness of disease-modifying therapies [15]. Nevertheless, caution is needed when interpreting the data, as neurofilament levels can increase with age [16]. This is particularly critical in identifying patients at risk of developing progressive forms of the disease, which are more prevalent in older individuals. There is a positive correlation between serum and CSF levels of neurofilaments [17], which is an advantage since lumbar puncture is a more invasive procedure.

Omics have been used for increasing the portfolio of putative biomarkers for MS, allowing not only a differential diagnostic but also predictive, prognostic, and therapeutic. Once different types of molecules are intricate in MS, some hallmarks of omics can be highlighted (**Figure 3**).

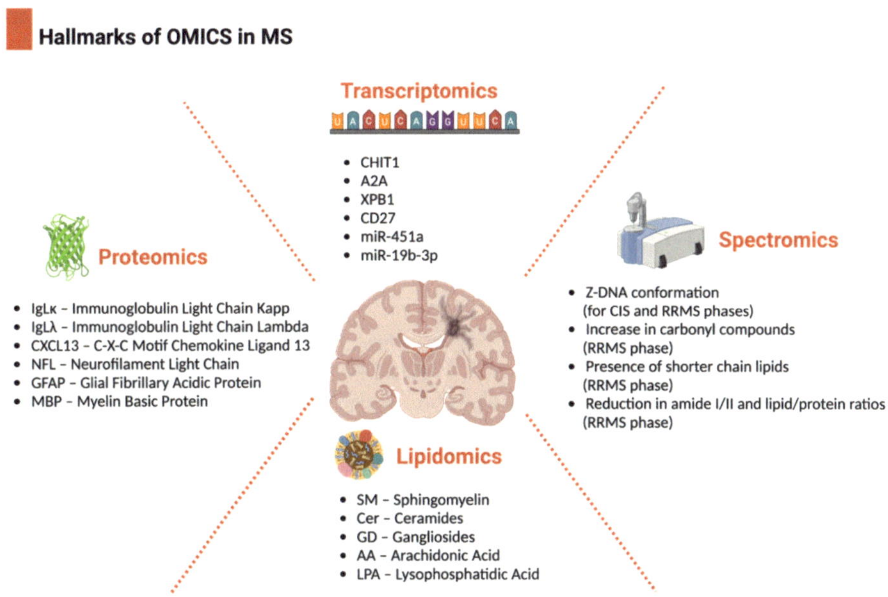

Figure 3.
Multi-omics hallmarks and the main findings related to multiple sclerosis biomarkers.

3. Transcriptomic of CSF

Transcriptomics is a technology based on the study of multiple RNA molecules, having tissue, whole blood or other fluids such as CSF used as matrices. This technique allows the evaluation of different RNAs under specific physiological aspects and different types of stimuli (chemical, physical) resulting from homeostasis or problems in the biological system. Although it has been widely used in cancer research, there are few studies in MS, leaving several questions still unanswered. Depending on the research objective, different methods can be used to study the transcriptome, including RNA sequencing (RNA-seq), its single-cell variant (scRNA-seq), microarrays, and reverse transcription-quantitative polymerase chain reaction (RT-qPCR). The gene expression analysis using scRNA-seq is particularly useful for characterizing cell lineages and phenotypes, and most studies investigate the expression of immune and brain cells present in the CSF of patients with MS, focusing on better understanding the basis of disease's pathophysiology [18–21]. On the other hand, RNA-seq, microarray, and RT-qPCR analysis are more commonly employed to discover potential diagnostic, prognostic, and predictive biomarkers, which is particularly convenient, since RNA molecules are small enough to cross the blood-brain barrier (BBB) into the CSF and provide useful information about the brain microenvironment [22–24].

The RT-qPCR is a popular technique for measuring the expression of both mRNAs and non-coding RNAs. Due to its high precision, specificity and relatively low cost, RT-qPCR is commonly employed to validate transcriptomic data based on reference genes. However, it is not capable of identifying novel transcripts across the whole transcriptome, and the number of genes tested per experiment is limited [25, 26]. In the context of MS patients, a study using CSF to identify diagnostic biomarkers capable of distinguishing MS and Neuro-Behçet's disease (NBD) from healthy controls, and from each other, revealed a set of five genes IL-17, IFN-γ, A2A, IL-1β, and CD39 with significance in differentiating patients with both diseases from healthy controls. However, differentiation between MS and NBD expression was not observed [23]. As potential diagnostic biomarkers for relapsing-remitting MS (RRMS), some microRNAs (miRNAs) such as Let-7g-5p, miR-18a-5p, miR-145-5p, miR-374a-5p, miR-150-5p, and miR-342-3p were identified in both CSF and blood exosomes [27].

The application of microarray technology in the field of transcriptomics offers advantages such as the ability to test a large number of genes in a single experiment and its well-established use in clinical practice. In summary, a chip can simultaneously assess the expression of thousands of genes on a small silica or glass slide [28, 29]. A microarray analysis performed in CSF of patients with MS revealed a set of seven central genes (STK4, RB1, CDKN1A, CDK1, RAC1, EZH2, and SDCBP) associated with pathways such as immune response, apoptosis, cell cycle regulation, and cell adhesion. These genes demonstrated the potential to differentiate MS patients from healthy controls [30]. The analysis of gene expression datasets, combined with protein expression data, is also commonly employed in research to validate biomarkers. Li et al. [24] employed publicly available microarray data, in conjunction with experimental data from flow cytometry, to identify and validate extracellular proteins in CSF as diagnostic biomarkers for RRMS, given their secretion into body fluids. After the analysis, Del-1 was proposed as a molecule of interest.

Among the methods mentioned here, RNA-seq is the only technique capable of discovering novel transcripts. It also offers the highest resolution, at the nucleotide level, and the broadest dynamic range for detecting gene expression [31, 32]. Despite the inherent fragility of RNA molecules, significant levels of mRNAs and non-coding RNAs in CSF were associated with the MS pathophysiology, which might not be replicable in the blood. The study of non-coding RNAs is particularly valuable for uncovering molecular regulatory mechanisms underlying the disease, as well as its clinical phenotypes. Among the different types of non-coding RNA, seven miRNAs exhibited differential expression levels in MS patients (miR-451a, miR-16-2-3p, miR-9-5p, miR-15a-5p, miR-144-3p, miR-100-5p, and miR-210-3p). They were enough to distinguish the RRMS phase from the progressive phase, potentially reflecting a shift toward a more neurodegenerative and less inflammatory disease profile. Based on this, RNA-seq analysis has shown that the miRNA profiles in blood samples differ from those in CSF, with the latter showing a stronger association with brain tissue cells. If these associations can be validated in large cohorts, the quantification of these molecules may be a valuable tool for diagnostic or prognostic purposes [22].

Finally, scRNA-seq, a variation of RNA-seq that assesses the expression profile of a single cell, has also been applied in studies in MS using CSF [33]. Its ability to provide detailed information about the cell types responsible for initiating and sustaining pathological stimuli makes it particularly valuable for investigating a disease with an undefined pathogenesis. Comparing the transcriptional composition of leukocytes in different matrices (blood and CSF) and in CSF under homeostatic (control) and inflammatory (MS) conditions, distinct compositions were found. The CSF exhibited to be enriched in T regulatory (Treg) cells, as well as cells of the myeloid (mDC1) and monocytic (Mono 2) lineages. These cells express specific markers associated with perivascular macrophages, CNS-border-associated macrophages, and resident macrophages. The scRNA-seq also identified an inflammatory expression signature, indicative of CNS tissue damage, characterized by the upregulation of molecules involved in chemokine signaling, lipid antigen recognition, and antigen presentation [18]. In fact, a similar inflammatory profile was confirmed in other studies. One highlights the role of CD8+ T cells and mDC1 in the CSF, driven by type 1 IFN response and regulated by genes such as ZC3HAV1 and IFITM2, suggesting a general dysregulation of antiviral mechanisms in MS [19]. The other one identified two clusters of expression, one of which was associated with immunoglobulin synthesis and protein production, marked by the expression of CD27 and XBP1, and another related to mitotic division and cytoskeleton organization, evidenced by MK167. Despite these distinctions, both clusters likely represent the same clonal lineage at different stages of maturation [20]. Cytokines, chemokines, and their receptors were also groups of genes highly expressed [21].

In the field of predictive biomarkers for MS progression, the investigation of CSF using scRNA-seq combined with post-mortem brain analysis reinforced the relevance of five myeloid markers in myeloid activation and their potential prognostic value. Among them, CHIT1 was identified as a strong candidate for predicting faster disability progression in MS due to its predominant expression in microglia located in active lesions. Its expression levels were correlated with microglial activity during disease progression [34]. To explore potential therapeutic targets for drug repositioning in MS, a study using CSF and blood samples identified several immunological pathways and screened pharmacological compounds that inhibit these processes, showing mTOR, PIK3, and HSP90 as promising therapeutic targets. Among the identified molecules, luminespib, an HSP90 inhibitor, was found to target all cell types identified in peripheral blood mononuclear cells (PBMC) and CSF. Another medicine, mitoxantrone, showed a strong association with the transcriptional reversion of most cell types and was approved for clinical use by the FDA [35], although this medication is rarely used due to its considerable cardiotoxic potential and the availability of safer medications.

4. Proteomic

Proteomics allows the identification of protein profiles associated with specific conditions, showing biological relevance once these molecules perform multiple and essential functions in the human body [36]. In this context, advances in proteomics have paved the understanding of the molecular mechanisms underlying MS, with some studies focusing on the identification of biomarkers for diagnosis, disease progression assessment, and therapeutic response evaluation [37]. This approach improved the translational science, bringing the OCBs [38], kappa, and lambda immunoglobulin light chains as key parameters for MS diagnosis, once they were overexpressed in MS and reflected an exacerbated intrathecal antibody production and intense B-cell-mediated inflammatory activity [39]. The neurofilament light chain (NFL), glial fibrillary acidic protein (GFAP), and myelin basic protein (MBP) are also used as indicators of axonal injury, astrocyte damage, and myelin degradation, respectively [40–42].

Proteomics revealed inflammatory biomarkers such as CXCL13, IL-6, and IL-8 associated with inflammatory activity and MS progression [43, 44]. These mediators play a crucial role in identifying the immunological stimuli characteristic of the disease. Beyond this, some biomarkers were correlated with established clinical evaluation criteria, such as the Expanded Disability Status Scale (EDSS). A notable example is chitinase-3-like protein 1 (YKL-40), a glycoprotein secreted by reactive astrocytes, which has been linked to exacerbate cerebral inflammation. Studies indicate that YKL-40 exhibits a positive correlation with higher EDSS scores, reflecting greater functional impairment. Furthermore, this protein is particularly prominent in the progressive phenotype of MS, where it is associated with neurodegeneration and gradual accumulation of disability [45]. These findings, encompassing both those already applied in clinical practice and those under investigation, holding the potential as complementary parameters for MS assessment. Moreover, they can contribute to the algorithms designed to identify disease-specific patterns and validate novel biomarkers.

5. Lipidomic

Beyond the study of proteins, an emerging molecular approach is lipidomics. In the context of MS, the importance of lipidomics arises from the central role of lipid metabolism in maintaining CNS health, particularly in the synthesis of the myelin sheath, a pivotal structure to the disease's pathophysiology. Moreover, lipids are key regulators of inflammatory pathways implicated in the pathogenesis of MS [46].

Comprehensive CSF lipidomics has demonstrated the ability to identify lipid clusters that distinguish MS patients from non-MS individuals using supervised methods. A notable upregulation of glycerophospholipids, associated with lipid pathways, was found implicated in MS pathophysiology [47]. Lysophosphatidic acid (LPA), a bioactive lipid alongside the biosynthesis of phospholipids, is released by inflammatory cells and neurons. It also showed to be of interest, once it is elevated in patients during relapses compared to those in remission. On the other hand, reduced LPA levels in CSF have been identified following pharmacological treatment. This behavior points out LPA as a potential marker of disease activity and also a biomarker for monitoring therapeutic responses [48].

Some evidence also suggests that the arachidonic acid pathway is hyperactivated during inflammatory states in MS, being released through the action of phospholipases on phospholipid membranes. The phospholipase activation has been associated with tumor necrosis factor-alpha (TNF-α), a cytokine abundantly present in inflammatory processes, that leads to the release of arachidonic acid and the subsequent activation of sphingomyelinases [49]. These enzymes initiate the breakdown of sphingomyelin, an essential component of CNS cell membranes that, along with alterations in gangliosides, may directly reflect demyelination processes. Preliminary studies indicate an increase in these molecules in CSF, along with elevated ceramide levels, which have been linked to axonal damage and mitochondrial dysfunction. Ceramides can promote the generation of reactive oxygen species (ROS), exacerbating oxidative stress in the CNS. Such lipid profiles hold therapeutic potential, once specific lipid metabolic pathways have been associated with remyelination processes [47]. Additionally, demyelination alters the intrathecal lipid composition. The disruption of the BBB further contributes to this by allowing the influx of circulating lipids into the CSF. These changes result in alterations in both absolute and relative quantities of lipids in individuals with BBB dysfunction. Although significant, changes in the CSF lipid profile are not exclusive to MS, and have also been observed in other neurodegenerative diseases, such as Guillain-Barré syndrome [50]. Therefore, the analysis for potential lipid markers must be integrated with the clinical presentation to achieve diagnostic precision.

6. Spectromics

In the last decades, methodologies using infrared spectroscopy with Fourier transform (FTIR) combined with chemometric techniques have been widely developed and applied in scientific research for diagnostic related to diseases with neurological impact, such as zika, COVID-19 [51–54], and some autoimmune diseases [55], among others.

This method is based on the measurement of the infrared region of the electromagnetic radiation spectrum [56]. The range comprising 3600–1250 cm^{-1}, called the group frequency region, is characterized by specific absorption bands associated with the fundamental vibrations of functional groups present in molecules, such as stretching of O−H, N−H, C−H, C=O, among others [57]. These bands are less influenced by interactions between different parts of the molecule, making them useful for identifying the presence of certain chemical groups. By another hand, in the spectral range between 1200 and 600 cm^{-1}, small variations in molecular structure and composition generate highly specific absorption bands for each molecule, due to the complex vibrations resulting from interactions between different chemical bonds. This range is extremely useful for accurately identifying and differentiating chemical compounds and is therefore called the fingerprint region [58]. In biofluid analysis, generally, the most relevant region ranges from 180 to 900 cm^{-1}, recognized as the "bio-fingerprint" region, where absorption peaks referring to the vibrations of functional groups present in proteins, lipids, carbohydrates and nucleic acids (DNA and RNA) [59, 60].

FTIR spectrometers allow the simultaneous acquisition of all frequencies, presenting high sensitivity, signal-to-noise ratio, and resolution. In addition, it is easy to use, and speed analysis characteristics [58] make FTIR an attractive approach for screening. Combined with the operating mode based on attenuated total reflectance (ATR), the technique also has the advantages of being non-destructive, suitable for solids, liquids, pastes, and thin films, with little or no sample preparation, regardless of its thickness [59]. Then, FTIR-ATR can be advantageous in the context of biofluid analysis [61–64], able to characterize spectral changes caused by different diseases once pathological conditions are associated with significant functional and structural changes in biological systems.

In this sense, FTIR-ATR spectroscopy was successfully used in CSF samples in the development of diagnostic methodology for patients with MS, as well as in the differential diagnosis between RRMS and CIS [65]. The evaluation of CSF from these patients and control samples, collected from patients treated for orthopedic problems but not diagnosed with neurological problems, showed that FTIR-ATR was capable of clustering the groups of MS patients apart of the negative controls, mainly in the spectral bands which correspond to the C-H vibrations, associated with lipid spectral bands and related to the conformation of Z-DNA. In advance, this data was used to perform a model for classifying MS patients. Together with a soft independent modeling of class analogy (SIMCA) classification, the model applied to 15 CIS samples was able to predict 10 samples as RRMS, a result confirmed 24 months later in a follow-up period. It suggests its potential for early diagnosis of RRMS, which could enable accurate treatment for delaying the conversion of CIS patients into RRMS ones. It is important to note that it is an incipient methodology, which requires more research, standardization of sample collection and processing protocols, and greater numbers of samples belonging to different groups of MS patients. Then, a truly robust and effective model can be built for the diagnosis of MS and identification of the stages of disease progression.

7. Conclusion

Multiple sclerosis remains a challenging and disabling condition, occurring in a "black box" hardly accessible, which avoids a clear comprehension of the disease triggers and the mechanisms of brain response to its biochemical impairment. The improvement in omics fields is helping to overcome some of these barriers, bringing to light biomarkers in the cerebrospinal fluid that represent the physiological conditions in the brain. In order to achieve successful results, it is important to combine clinical and multi-omics data, selecting the best strategy to be used as clinical support, assuring better clinical intervention and promoting life quality for the patients.

Conflict of interest

The authors declare no conflict of interest.

Author details

Kleiton de Barros Borges[1,2,3], Victória Regina da Silva[1], Jordana Marina da Silva[1], Valéria Visani[1], Maria Helena Menezes Estevam Alves[1]
and Danyelly Bruneska Gondim Martins[1,4]*

1 Keizo Asami Institute (iLIKA), Federal University of Pernambuco, Brazil

2 Oswaldo Cruz Hospital, University of Pernambuco, Brazil

3 Department of Neurology, Royal Portuguese Hospital, Pernambuco, Brazil

4 Department of Biochemistry, Federal University of Pernambuco, Brazil

*Address all correspondence to: bruneska@prospecmol.org

References

[1] International Multiple Sclerosis Genetics Consortium (IMSGC), Beecham AH, Patsopoulos NA, Xifara DK, Davis MF, Kemppinen A, et al. Analysis of immune-related loci identifies 48 new susceptibility variants for multiple sclerosis. Nature Genetics. 2013;**45**(11):1353-1360. DOI: 10.1038/ng.2770. Epub 2013 Sep 29

[2] Thompson AJ, Banwell BL, Barkhof F, Carroll WM, Coetzee T, Comi G, et al. Diagnosis of multiple sclerosis: 2017 revisions of the McDonald criteria. Lancet Neurology. 2018;**17**(2):162-173. DOI: 10.1016/S1474-4422(17)30470-2. Epub 2017 Dec 21

[3] Tintore M, Rovira À, Río J, Otero-Romero S, Arrambide G, Tur C, et al. Defining high, medium and low impact prognostic factors for developing multiple sclerosis. Brain. 2015;**138**(Pt 7):1863-1874. DOI: 10.1093/brain/awv105. Epub 2015 Apr 21

[4] Bielekova B, Martin R. Development of biomarkers in multiple sclerosis. Brain. 2004;**127**(Pt 7):1463-1478. DOI: 10.1093/brain/awh176. Epub 2004 Jun 4

[5] Sellebjerg F, Börnsen L, Ammitzbøll C, Nielsen JE, Vinther-Jensen T, Hjermind LE, et al. Defining active progressive multiple sclerosis. Multiple Sclerosis. 2017;**23**(13):1727-1735. DOI: 10.1177/1352458517726592. Epub 2017 Aug 23

[6] Freedman MS, Thompson EJ, Deisenhammer F, Giovannoni G, Grimsley G, Keir G, et al. Recommended standard of cerebrospinal fluid analysis in the diagnosis of multiple sclerosis: A consensus statement. Archives of Neurology. 2005;**62**(6):865-870. DOI: 10.1001/archneur.62.6.865

[7] Arrambide G, Tintore M, Espejo C, Auger C, Castillo M, Río J, et al. The value of oligoclonal bands in the multiple sclerosis diagnostic criteria. Brain. 2018;**141**(4):1075-1084. DOI: 10.1093/brain/awy006

[8] Gastaldi M, Zardini E, Leante R, Ruggieri M, Costa G, Cocco E, et al. Cerebrospinal fluid analysis and the determination of oligoclonal bands. Neurological Sciences. 2017;**38**(Suppl 2):217-224. DOI: 10.1007/s10072-017-3034-2

[9] Altıokka-Uzun G, Tüzün E, Ekizoğlu E, Ulusoy C, Yentür S, Kürtüncü M, et al. Oligoclonal bands and increased cytokine levels in idiopathic intracranial hypertension. Cephalalgia. 2015;**35**(13):1153-1161. DOI: 10.1177/0333102415570762. Epub 2015 Feb 19

[10] Jarius S, Paul F, Franciotta D, Ruprecht K, Ringelstein M, Bergamaschi R, et al. Cerebrospinal fluid findings in aquaporin-4 antibody positive neuromyelitis optica: Results from 211 lumbar punctures. Journal of the Neurological Sciences. 2011;**306**(1-2):82-90. DOI: 10.1016/j.jns.2011.03.038. Epub 2011 May 6

[11] Jarius S, Pellkofer H, Siebert N, Korporal-Kuhnke M, Hümmert MW, Ringelstein M, et al. Cerebrospinal fluid findings in patients with myelin oligodendrocyte glycoprotein (MOG) antibodies. Part 1: Results from 163 lumbar punctures in 100 adult patients. Journal of Neuroinflammation. 2020;**17**(1):261. DOI: 10.1186/s12974-020-01824-2

[12] Hegen H, Berek K, Deisenhammer F. Cerebrospinal fluid kappa free light

chains as biomarker in multiple sclerosis-from diagnosis to prediction of disease activity. Wiener Medizinische Wochenschrift. 2022;**172**(15-16):337-345. DOI: 10.1007/s10354-022-00912-7. Epub 2022 Feb 8

[13] Hegen H, Arrambide G, Gnanapavan S, Kaplan B, Khalil M, Saadeh R, et al. Cerebrospinal fluid kappa free light chains for the diagnosis of multiple sclerosis: A consensus statement. Multiple Sclerosis. 2023;**29**(2):182-195. DOI: 10.1177/13524585221134217. Epub 2022 Dec 17

[14] Wang H, Wu M, Zhan C, Ma E, Yang M, Yang X, et al. Neurofilament proteins in axonal regeneration and neurodegenerative diseases. Neural Regeneration Research. 2012;**7**(8):620-626. DOI: 10.3969/j.issn.1673-5374.2012.08.010

[15] Freedman MS, Gnanapavan S, Booth RA, Calabresi PA, Khalil M, Kuhle J, et al. Guidance for use of neurofilament light chain as a cerebrospinal fluid and blood biomarker in multiple sclerosis management. eBioMedicine. 2024;**101**:104970. DOI: 10.1016/j.ebiom.2024.104970

[16] Kapoor R, Smith KE, Allegretta M, Arnold DL, Carroll W, Comabella M, et al. Serum neurofilament light as a biomarker in progressive multiple sclerosis. Neurology. 2020;**95**(10):436-444. DOI: 10.1212/WNL.0000000000010346

[17] Novakova L, Zetterberg H, Sundström P, Axelsson M, Khademi M, Gunnarsson M, et al. Monitoring disease activity in multiple sclerosis using serum neurofilament light protein. Neurology. 2017;**89**(22):2230-2237. DOI: 10.1212/WNL.0000000000004683

[18] Schafflick D et al. Integrated single cell analysis of blood and cerebrospinal fluid leukocytes in multiple sclerosis. Nature Communications. 2020;**11**(1):247. DOI: 10.1038/s41467-019-14118-w

[19] Ban M, Bredikhin D, Huang Y, Bonder MJ, Katarzyna K, Oliver AJ, et al. Expression profiling of cerebrospinal fluid identifies dysregulated antiviral mechanisms in multiple sclerosis. Brain. 2024;**147**(2):554-565. DOI: 10.1093/brain/awad404

[20] Polak J et al. Single-cell transcriptomics combined with proteomics of intrathecal IgG reveal transcriptional heterogeneity of oligoclonal IgG-secreting cells in multiple sclerosis. Frontiers in Cellular Neuroscience. 2023;**17**:01-07. DOI: 10.3389/fncel.2023.1189709

[21] Ramesh A et al. A pathogenic and clonally expanded B cell transcriptome in active multiple sclerosis. Proceedings of the National Academy of Sciences. 2020;**117**(37):22932-22943. DOI: 10.1073/pnas.2008523117

[22] Tan IL et al. Potential biomarkers for multiple sclerosis stage from targeted proteomics and microRNA sequencing. Brain Communications. 2024;**6**(4):01-18. DOI: 10.1093/braincomms/fcae209

[23] Maghrebi O et al. Differential gene expression patterns in blood and cerebrospinal fluid of multiple sclerosis and Neuro-Behçet disease. Frontiers in Genetics. 2021;**12**:01-11. DOI: 10.3389/fgene.2021.638236

[24] Li M et al. Identification and clinical validation of key extracellular proteins as the potential biomarkers in relapsing-remitting multiple sclerosis. Frontiers in Immunology. 2021;**12**:01-14. DOI: 10.3389/fimmu.2021.753929

[25] Bong D, Sohn J, Lee S-JV. Brief guide to RT-qPCR. Molecules and Cells. 2024;**47**(12):100141. DOI: 10.1016/j.mocell.2024.100141

[26] De Brito MWD et al. RNA-seq validation: Software for selection of reference and variable candidate genes for RT-qPCR. BMC Genomics. 2024;**25**(1):697. DOI: 10.1186/s12864-024-10511-y

[27] Mohammadinasr M et al. Multiplex analysis of cerebrospinal fluid and serum exosomes MicroRNAs of untreated relapsing remitting multiple sclerosis (RRMS) and proposing noninvasive diagnostic biomarkers. Neuromolecular Medicine. 2023;**25**(3):402-414. DOI: 10.1007/s12017-023-08744-3

[28] Govindarajan R et al. Microarray and its applications. Journal of Pharmacy and Bioallied Sciences. 2012;**4**(6):310. DOI: 10.4103/0975-7406.100283

[29] Greenberg SA. DNA microarray gene expression analysis technology and its application to neurological disorders. Neurology. 2001;**57**(5):755-761. DOI: 10.1212/WNL.57.5.755

[30] Safari-Alighiarloo N et al. Network-based analysis of differentially expressed genes in cerebrospinal fluid (CSF) and blood reveals new candidate genes for multiple sclerosis. PeerJ. 2016;**4**:e2775. DOI: 10.7717/peerj.2775

[31] Rodríguez-García A, Sola-Landa A, Barreiro C. RNA Preparation and RNA-Seq Bioinformatics for Comparative Transcriptomics. Methods in Molecular Biology. 2023;**2704**:99-113. DOI: 10.1007/978-1-0716-3385-4_6

[32] Wang Z, Gerstein M, Snyder M. RNA-Seq: A revolutionary tool for transcriptomics. Nature Reviews Genetics. 2009;**10**(1):57-63. DOI: 10.1038/nrg2484

[33] Haque A et al. A practical guide to single-cell RNA-sequencing for biomedical research and clinical applications. Genome Medicine. 2017;**9**(1):75. DOI: 10.1186/s13073-017-0467-4

[34] Belien J et al. CHIT1 at diagnosis predicts faster disability progression and reflects early microglial activation in multiple sclerosis. Nature Communications. 2024;**15**(1):5013. DOI: 10.1038/s41467-024-49312-y

[35] Shevtsov A et al. In silico drug repurposing in multiple sclerosis using scRNA-Seq data. International Journal of Molecular Sciences. 2023;**24**(2):985. DOI: 10.3390/ijms24020985

[36] Veenstra TD. Omics in systems biology: Current progress and future outlook. Proteomics. 2021;**21**(3-4):2000235. DOI: 10.1002/pmic.202000235

[37] Yang J et al. Current and future biomarkers in multiple sclerosis. International Journal of Molecular Sciences. 2022;**23**(11):5877. DOI: 10.3390/ijms23115877

[38] Maglio G et al. Multiple sclerosis: From the application of oligoclonal bands to novel potential biomarkers. International Journal of Molecular Sciences. 2024;**25**(10):5412. DOI: 10.3390/ijms25105412

[39] Arneth B, Kraus J. The use of kappa free light chains to diagnose multiple sclerosis. Medicina. 2022;**58**(11):1512. DOI: 10.3390/medicina58111512

[40] Ferreira-Atuesta C et al. The evolution of neurofilament light chain in multiple sclerosis. Frontiers in Neuroscience. 2021;**15**:642384. DOI: 10.3389/fnins.2021.642384

[41] Jiang X et al. Glial fibrillary acidic protein and multiple sclerosis progression independent of acute inflammation. Multiple Sclerosis Journal. 2023;**29**(9):1070-1079. DOI: 10.1177/13524585231176732

[42] Agliardi C et al. Myelin basic protein in oligodendrocyte-derived extracellular vesicles as a diagnostic and prognostic biomarker in multiple sclerosis: A pilot study. International Journal of Molecular Sciences. 2023;**24**(1):894. DOI: 10.3390/ijms24010894

[43] Pancher AR et al. CXCL13 as a biomarker: Background and utility in multiple sclerosis. Biomolecules. 2024;**14**(12):1541. DOI: 10.3390/biom14121541

[44] Alrafiah A et al. Expression patterns of inflammatory cytokines in multiple sclerosis patients. Tropical Journal of Pharmaceutical Research. 2024;**23**(10):1647-1652. DOI: 10.4314/tjpr.v23i10.8

[45] Talaat F et al. Chitinase-3-like 1-protein in CSF: A novel biomarker for progression in patients with multiple sclerosis. Neurological Sciences. 2023;**44**(9):3243-3252. DOI: 10.1007/s10072-023-06764-2

[46] Castellanos DB et al. Brain lipidomics as a rising field in neurodegenerative contexts: Perspectives with machine learning approaches. Frontiers in Neuroendocrinology. 2021;**61**:100899. DOI: 10.1016/j.yfrne.2021.100899

[47] Oliveira EMLD et al. Multiple sclerosis has a distinct lipid signature in plasma and cerebrospinal fluid. Arquivos de Neuro-Psiquiatria. 2019;**77**:696-704. DOI: 10.1590/0004-282X20190122

[48] Jiang D et al. Elevated lysophosphatidic acid levels in the serum and cerebrospinal fluid in patients with multiple sclerosis: Therapeutic response and clinical implication. Neurological Research. 2018;**40**(5):335-339. DOI: 10.1080/01616412.2018.1446256

[49] Ferreira HB et al. An overview of lipidomic analysis in different human matrices of multiple sclerosis. Multiple Sclerosis and Related Disorders. 2020;**44**:102189. DOI: 10.1016/j.msard.2020.102189

[50] Péter M et al. Cerebrospinal fluid lipidomic biomarker signatures of demyelination for multiple sclerosis and Guillain–Barré syndrome. Scientific Reports. 2020;**10**(1):18380. DOI: 10.1038/s41598-020-75502-x

[51] Barauna VG et al. Ultrarapid on-site detection of SARS-CoV-2 infection using simple ATR-FTIR spectroscopy and an analysis algorithm: High sensitivity and specificity. Analytical Chemistry. 2021;**93**(5):2950-2958. DOI: 10.1021/acs.analchem.0c04608

[52] Nascimento MHC et al. Noninvasive diagnostic for COVID-19 from saliva biofluid via FTIR spectroscopy and multivariate analysis. Analytical Chemistry. 2022;**94**(5):2425-2433. DOI: 10.1021/acs.analchem.1c04162

[53] Nogueira MS et al. Rapid diagnosis of COVID-19 using FT-IR ATR spectroscopy and machine learning. Scientific Reports. 2021;**11**(1):1-13. DOI: 10.1038/s41598-021-93511-2

[54] Santos MCD et al. ATR-FTIR spectroscopy with chemometric algorithms of multivariate classification in the discrimination between healthy: Vs. dengue vs. chikungunya vs. zika clinical samples. Analytical Methods. 2018;**10**:1280-1285. DOI: 10.1039/C7AY02784B

[55] Alkhuder K. Fourier-transform infrared spectroscopy: A universal optical sensing technique with auspicious application prospects in the diagnosis and management of autoimmune diseases. Photodiagnosis and Photodynamic Therapy. 2023;**42**:103606. DOI: 10.1016/j.pdpdt.2023.103606

[56] Coates J. Interpretation of infrared spectra: A practical approach. In: Meyers RA, editor. Encyclopedia of Analytical Chemistry. Chichester: John Wiley & Sons Ltd.; 2000. pp. 10881-10882

[57] Pavia DL et al. Introduction to spectroscopy. 4th ed. Belmont, USA: Brooks/Cole Cengage Learning; 2009. p. 708. Library of Congress Control Number: 2007943966. ISBN-10:0495114782; ISBN-13: 978-0495114789

[58] Holler FJ, Skoog DA, Crouch SR. Princípios de Análise Instrumental. 6th ed. Porto Alegre, Brazil: Bookman; 2009. ISBN-10:8577804607, ISBN-13:978-8577804603

[59] Mitchell AL et al. Vibrational spectroscopy of biofluids for disease screening or diagnosis: Translation from the laboratory to a clinical setting. Journal of Biophotonics. 2014;**7**(3-4):153-165. DOI: 10.1002/jbio.201400018

[60] Baker JM et al. Developing and understanding biofluid vibrational spectroscopy: A critical review. Chemical Society Reviews. 2015;**45**(7):1803-1818. DOI: 10.1039/C5CS00585J

[61] Rutherford SH, Nordon A, Hunt NT, Baker MJ. Biofluid analysis and classification using IR and 2D-IR spectroscopy. Chemometrics and Intelligent Laboratory Systems. 2021;**217**. DOI: 10.1016/j.chemolab.2021.104408

[62] Shaw RA, Mantsch HH. Infrared spectroscopy of biological fluids in clinical and diagnostic analysis. In: Meyers RA, Meyers RA, editors. Encyclopedia of Analytical Chemistry: Applications, Theory and Instrumentation. Wiley; 2008. DOI: 10.1002/9780470027318.a0106.pub2

[63] Leal LB, Nogueira MS, Canevari RA, Carvalho LFCS. Vibration spectroscopy and body biofluids: Literature review for clinical applications. Photodiagnosis and Photodynamic Therapy. 2018;**24**:237-244. DOI: 10.1016/j.pdpdt.2018.09.008

[64] Beć KB, Grabska J, Huck CW. Biomolecular and bioanalytical applications of infrared spectroscopy – A review. Analytica Chimica Acta. 2020;**1133**:150-177. DOI: 10.1016/j.aca.2020.04.015

[65] Yonar D, Ocek L, Tiftikcioglu BI, Zorlu Y, Severcan F. Relapsing-remitting multiple sclerosis diagnosis from cerebrospinal fluids via Fourier transform infrared spectroscopy coupled with multivariate analysis. Scientific Reports. 2018;**8**(1). DOI: 10.1038/s41598-018-19303-3

Chapter 4

Atypical Presentation or Variants of Multiple Sclerosis

Eleni Litsou

Abstract

Multiple sclerosis (MS) is a chronic inflammatory demyelinating disorder (DD) of the central nervous system (CNS), characterized by the presence of multifocal lesions, axonal degeneration, and reactive gliosis. Remyelination may occur, particularly in the early phases of lesion development, although its extent varies among individuals. Pathological studies have highlighted significant inter-individual differences in oligodendrocyte preservation and distinct mechanisms of demyelination, including T-cell/macrophage-mediated processes, antibody/complement-mediated injury, and primary oligodendrocyte damage. Beyond classical MS, several atypical variants—such as tumefactive MS, BCS, Schilder's diffuse sclerosis, Marburg's acute MS and Neuromyelitis Optica Spectrum Disorder (NMOSD), share core pathological features with MS while exhibiting unique distinguishing characteristics. NMOSD, for instance, is strongly associated with aquaporin-4 (AQP4) autoantibodies and primarily involves antibody/complement-mediated demyelination, whereas BCS is marked by oligodendrocyte dystrophy and a distinct "onion-bulb" pattern of myelin loss. Acute disseminated encephalomyelitis (ADEM) represents a related inflammatory demyelinating condition but typically lacks extensive, chronic demyelination. Understanding these rare MS variants provides crucial insights into the diverse pathogenic mechanisms underlying CNS demyelination. This chapter aims to comprehensively explore these atypical forms of MS, highlighting their distinctive clinical presentations, imaging features, and pathological characteristics to improve diagnostic accuracy and therapeutic approaches.

Keywords: multiple sclerosis, Tumefactive multiple sclerosis, Balo's concentric sclerosis, Marburg's acute multiple sclerosis, Devic's neuromyelits optica, Schilder's diffuse sclerosis, acute disseminated encephalomyelitis

1. Introduction

1.1 The atypical spectrum of multiple sclerosis

MS is a chronic inflammatory DD of the CNS, characterized by immune-mediated damage leading to demyelination, axonal degeneration, and gliosis. The classical form of MS, initially described by Charcot, presents with multiple, well-demarcated plaques within the white matter of the brain and spinal cord. However, atypical demyelinating conditions exist, often considered MS variants, which exhibit distinct clinical and pathological features. These include Marburg's acute MS, BCS, neuromyelitis optica spectrum disorder (NMOSD), and Schilder's diffuse sclerosis. Additionally, ADEM is regarded as a closely related disorder with overlapping characteristics.

Although these atypical MS forms share fundamental pathological mechanisms with classical MS, they also possess unique distinguishing features. NMOSD, for instance, is characterized by antibody/complement-mediated demyelination, particularly targeting AQP4 in astrocytes. In contrast, BCS is associated with oligodendrocyte dystrophy and the formation of distinctive concentric rings of myelin loss and preservation. ADEM typically lacks chronic and extensive demyelination.

Recent research highlights the heterogeneity of demyelinating mechanisms underlying these MS variants, suggesting that multiple pathogenic pathways may contribute to disease progression. Studying these rare and atypical forms provides valuable insights into the broader spectrum of MS pathology, helping refine diagnostic criteria and improve therapeutic strategies tailored to specific demyelinating processes.

1.2 Pseudotumoral demyelinating lesions

Tumefactive demyelination (TD) is characterized by large, inflammatory demyelinating lesions within the CNS, often mimicking neoplastic processes. These tumefactive demyelinating lesions (TDLs) are generally defined as focal areas of demyelination exceeding 2 cm in diameter and may present as single or multiple lesions, predominantly affecting the cerebral white matter, brainstem, or cerebellum. While these lesions are frequently associated with MS (including TDLs, BCS, Schilder's sclerosis, and Marburg disease), they can also manifest independently or as part of various other DDs. Conditions such as NMOSD, myelin oligodendrocyte glycoprotein (MOG) antibody-associated demyelination (MOG-AD), ADEM, and acute hemorrhagic leukoencephalitis (AHLE) have all been reported to present with similar pathological features [1].

Their exact prevalence remains uncertain, though estimates suggest approximately three cases per million people [2], with an incidence ranging between 1.4% and 8.2% among individuals with MS [1]. Due to their appearance, pseudotumoral lesions may be misdiagnosed as abscesses or malignant tumors, potentially leading to unnecessary and risky brain biopsies, as well as delays in accurate diagnosis and appropriate treatment. Careful monitoring of both biopsied and non-biopsied lesions is essential once a diagnosis has been determined. Testing for AQP4-IgG and MOG-IgG is advisable when these lesions are identified. Magnetic resonance imaging (MRI) findings, particularly dynamic restricted diffusion at lesion borders, can help differentiate atypical demyelination from other possible conditions. Histopathological analysis suggests that tissue hypoxia might play a role in their development. CT-PET imaging can further assist in distinguishing pseudotumoral demyelination from high-grade tumors. Once malignancy is ruled out, uncertainties remain regarding the specific DD involved, as treatment approaches and long-term outlooks vary between MS and other related conditions. Current recommendations suggest that patients who meet the criteria for MS should receive standard treatments for the disease. Many individuals with pseudotumoral demyelinating lesions are ultimately diagnosed with MS. Some may experience a single episode or later be identified with NMOSD, MOG antibody-associated demyelination, or ADEM. Overall, understanding the diverse manifestations of tumefactive and pseudotumoral demyelination is crucial for timely diagnosis and appropriate management of affected individuals.

DOI: http://dx.doi.org/10.5772/intechopen.1010042

1.3 Tumefactive MS.

TDLs were initially documented by van der Velden et al. in 1979 [3]. These lesions are pathologically classified as an intermediary form between MS and ADEM plaques, which are two predominant types of CNS demyelinating diseases [4]. TD is a variant of MS characterized by large intracranial lesions resembling tumors, typically exceeding 2 cm in size. These lesions may present with cystic transformations or ring enhancement on MRI, exhibiting minimal edema and mass effect relative to lesion size [5, 6]. The lesion scan be singular or multiple and may emerge in any part of the CNS, including the spinal cord. Tumor-like demyelination in tumefactive MS is relatively uncommon, occurring in approximately 1–2 per 1000 MS cases or about 3 cases per million individuals annually. Although TDLs can manifest across different age groups, they are most commonly seen in young adults in their second or third decade of life, as previous studies have indicated [4, 7–9]. Additionally, a higher prevalence of TDLs has been observed in females, with a median onset age of 37 years [4].

The precise pathophysiological mechanisms underlying TDLs remain an area of ongoing investigation. Histopathological analyses reveal that these lesions are highly cellular, exhibiting extensive demyelination accompanied by an abundance of foamy macrophages laden with myelin debris. Reactive astrogliosis is a hallmark feature, while axonal structures remain relatively preserved. Varying degrees of perivascular and parenchymal lymphocytic infiltration are observed, suggesting an immune-mediated process (**Figure 1**). The prominent presence of macrophages and T lymphocytes within TDLs raises the possibility of a link to viral infections or vaccinations, similar to other demyelinating conditions [7–9].

One of the key clinical challenges associated with TDLs is their non-specific and often atypical presentation, particularly in tumefactive form, leading to frequent diagnostic dilemmas and delayed treatment initiation. Due to their size and imaging characteristics, TDLs are frequently mistaken for brain neoplasms rather than being immediately recognized as demyelinating lesions. The clinical symptoms vary but

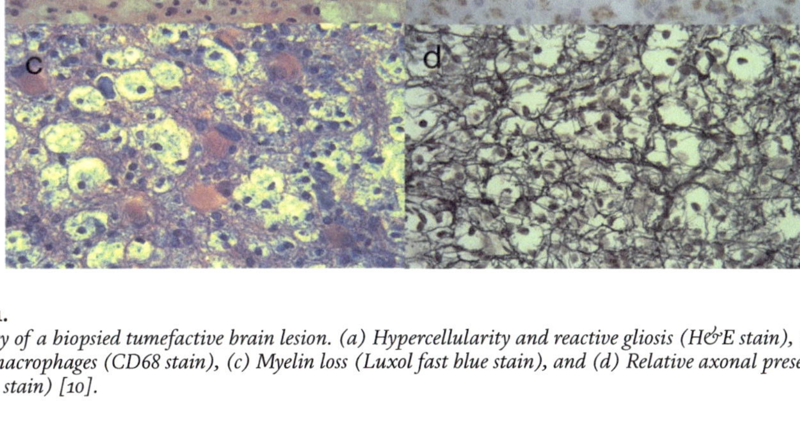

Figure 1.
Pathology of a biopsied tumefactive brain lesion. (a) Hypercellularity and reactive gliosis (H&E stain), (b) Foamy macrophages (CD68 stain), (c) Myelin loss (Luxol fast blue stain), and (d) Relative axonal preservation (Bodian stain) [10].

often include signs of increased intracranial pressure, such as persistent headaches, nausea, and vomiting. In some cases, patients present with focal neurological deficits, including hemiplegia and aphasia, or experience seizures, further complicating the differential diagnosis [2].

The interval between symptom onset and hospital admission varies depending on the clinical manifestation. Patients presenting with signs of increased intracranial pressure or focal neurological impairment typically seek medical attention within days to weeks, whereas those with seizures may remain undiagnosed for months or even years. Additional neurological symptoms associated with tumefactive MS include cognitive dysfunction, confusion, aphasia, apraxia, and seizure activity [4].

Diagnostic cerebrospinal fluid (CSF) analysis often reveals mild pleocytosis and slightly elevated protein concentrations, although oligoclonal bands are less frequently detected during the initial clinical episode compared to their prevalence in established MS (52% vs. 90%) [11]. This distinction underscores the need for careful diagnostic evaluation to differentiate TDLs from other DDs and space-occupying CNS lesions.

MRI serves as the primary imaging modality for diagnosing TDLs (**Figure 2**). However, these lesions pose a diagnostic dilemma due to their resemblance to gliomas when presenting as a solitary mass or to metastatic lesions when appearing as multiple separate foci [2, 4, 7–9, 13]. Distinct imaging characteristics have been identified to aid in differentiating TDLs from other CNS pathologies. Notable among these are the presence of ring-like or open-ring enhancement patterns and centrally dilated veins within the lesions [14–16]. In TDLs, contrast enhancement frequently manifests as

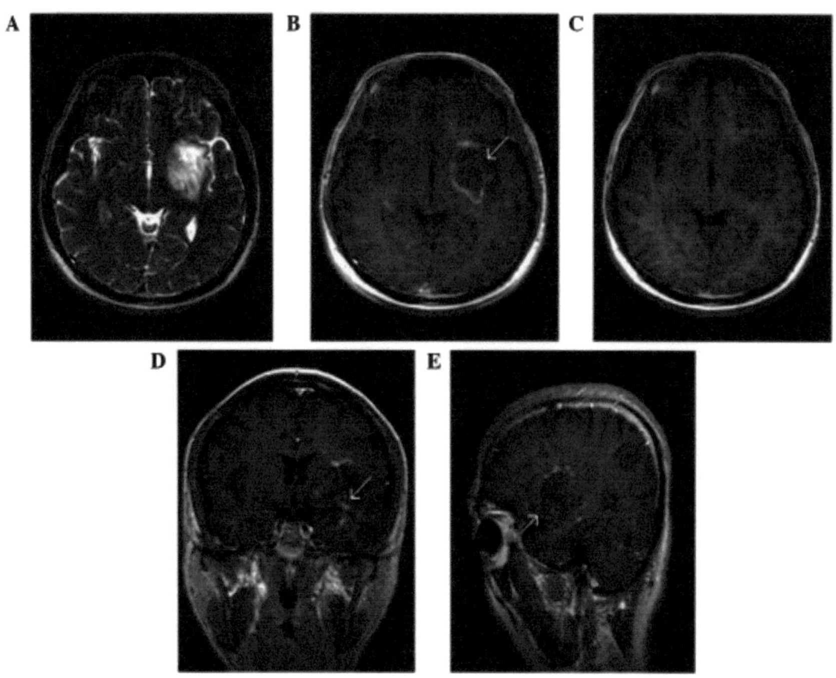

Figure 2.
MRI of a tumefactive demyelinating lesion. (A) Non-enhanced axial T2-weighted image showing a lesion in the left basal ganglia. (B) Enhanced axial T1-weighted image with ring-like enhancement. (C) Non-enhanced axial T1-weighted image. (D, E) Enhanced coronal T1-weighted images highlighting the lesion (arrows) [12].

an incomplete open ring, with the non-enhancing portion facing the gray matter. This feature is significantly more prevalent in TDLs, whereas it is observed in only approximately 9% of active MS plaques [17].

The contrast-enhancing segment of the ring is thought to indicate the advancing front of active demyelination predominantly occurring within the white matter, while the non-enhancing central region likely represents a chronic inflammatory phase. Additionally, these vascular structures have been linked to subependymal venous distension, with the dilated veins hypothesized to reflect an underlying disturbance in venous drainage [17–19].

Histopathological confirmation of TDLs can be complex, particularly when relying on frozen-section analysis, which may be insufficient for an accurate diagnosis [14]. The final diagnosis is typically determined through immunohistopathological examination. In clinical practice, TDLs are frequently misdiagnosed as gliomas due to their tumor-like characteristics [20]. Among brain tumors, gliomas are commonly confused with TDLs. High-grade gliomas, unlike TDLs, generally present with significant mass effect and extensive surrounding edema. Conversely, cerebral masses that demonstrate an acute or subacute onset, neurological deficits, ring-like enhancement with minimal mass effect, and limited surrounding edema on MRI should raise suspicion for TDLs.

Recognizing this MS variant is crucial, as these lesions are often subjected to biopsy or surgical resection due to diagnostic uncertainty, especially in small biopsy samples [4]. The histopathological features of TDLs can closely resemble neoplastic processes, leading to a significant challenge for neuropathologists. Inflammatory gliosis observed in active MS lesions can mimic the characteristics of glioblastoma, while the presence of inflammatory infiltrates may raise concerns for vasculitis, infectious etiologies, or lymphoproliferative disorders [21]. Given their hypercellular nature and presence of atypical reactive astrocytes and mitotic figures, biopsies of TDLs are frequently mistaken for neoplasms.

The prognosis and treatment of TDLs depend on the underlying demyelinating condition. Corticosteroids serve as the primary therapeutic approach [22]. Since most TDL patients respond well to corticosteroid therapy, surgical intervention is typically unnecessary. While some cases exhibit a diminished response to steroids, plasma exchange has been proposed as an alternative treatment [23–25]. Estimates suggest that within 45–70% of cases, a second clinical episode occurs within a median timeframe of 2–5 years [3, 26, 27].

1.4 Balò's concentric sclerosis

BCS is an uncommon DD that is considered a variant of MS. It is characterized by distinctive alternating bands of myelinated and demyelinated axons, creating a concentric, onion-like pattern on neuroimaging. The underlying mechanism of these concentric rings remains uncertain, though theories suggest they may represent either remyelination attempts or the early stages of demyelination. One hypothesis proposes that the formation of these rings begins with an initial core of demyelination, which becomes surrounded by an inflammatory ring acting as a protective barrier to prevent further expansion. As the disease progresses, this core breaches the protective ring, leading to the distinctive layered appearance seen in imaging studies [22].

Clinically, BCS presents with a highly variable neurological profile, depending on lesion location. Common symptoms include headaches, muscle weakness, seizures, aphasia, cognitive impairment, and sensory disturbances. Lesions may develop in multiple areas of the CNS, including the cerebral hemispheres, brainstem, cerebellum, spinal cord, and optic chiasm.

To date, there is a higher prevalence among males aged 4–56 years [28, 29]. Initially described in Central Europe, BCS has since been identified more frequently in Asian populations [30]. The disease can manifest in different clinical courses, ranging from a single, self-limited episode to a relapsing-remitting or primary progressive pattern. Historically, BCS was thought to lead to rapid neurological deterioration, resembling Marburg's acute MS. However, more recent studies suggest that some individuals experience extended survival, spontaneous remission, or only mild long-term deficits. Advances in early MRI detection and prompt corticosteroid therapy have contributed significantly to improved outcomes in affected patients [31].

The onset of BCS typically occurs between 20 and 50 years of age, with patients predominantly presenting with cerebral symptoms. Common initial manifestations include prodromal fever, headaches, and neurological deficits, with a noted predominance in female patients [32]. Distinct characteristics that set BCS apart from MS include its unique lesion morphology—defined by alternating layers of demyelinated and preserved myelin-forming a concentric "onion-like" pattern—along with a higher prevalence of large tumefactive lesions, a disease course that is often monophasic and self-limiting, and a severity that can sometimes lead to a fatal outcome in its first presentation. These distinctions suggest that BCS may represent a distinct pathophysiological entity [33].

The characteristic concentric lesions of BCS were first described by Otto Marburg in 1906 in cases of fulminant MS and later by Joseph Balò in 1927 [34]. While similar bands have been observed in some MS cases, BCS lesions appear to have a different pathophysiological mechanism. These lesions occur against a backdrop of T cell-mediated inflammation with significant macrophage and microglia activation. Several hypotheses have been proposed regarding their formation, including ischemia, remyelination processes, or the diffusion of myelin-toxic factors within the extracellular matrix. Recent research suggests that the development of concentric lesions may be driven by tissue preconditioning, induced by hypoxia-like injury, where stress-related proteins are upregulated to protect intact myelin against further damage in an expanding lesion [35]. In affected areas, increased expression of inducible nitric oxide synthase (i-NOS) has been identified, implicating oxidative stress and mitochondrial injury as potential contributors to disease progression.

Magnetic resonance imaging (MRI) is crucial in diagnosing BCS, as its hallmark concentric ring pattern is considered pathognomonic. These alternating bands of demyelination and preserved myelin create distinctive signal intensities on various MRI sequences [28, 36]. On T2-weighted images, active demyelinating areas appear hyperintense, interspersed with isointense bands corresponding to preserved myelin (**Figure 3A**). Similarly, on T1-weighted images, myelinated regions appear isointense, whereas demyelinated zones present as hypointense rings (**Figure 3B**). Gadolinium-enhanced T1-weighted images further reveal concentric ring enhancement at sites of increased blood-brain barrier permeability and inflammatory demyelination [38, 39]. Diffusion-weighted imaging (DWI) and diffusion coefficient mapping have further contributed to the characterization of BCS lesions. Areas of active demyelination exhibit restricted diffusion, appearing as hyperintense regions on DWI, whereas preserved or remyelinated areas display facilitated diffusion, appearing hypointense (**Figure 3G**). These imaging features aid in differentiating BCS from other demyelinating and neoplastic conditions. Restricted diffusion is initially localized around the lesion's central core and gradually extends outward, supporting the hypothesis that

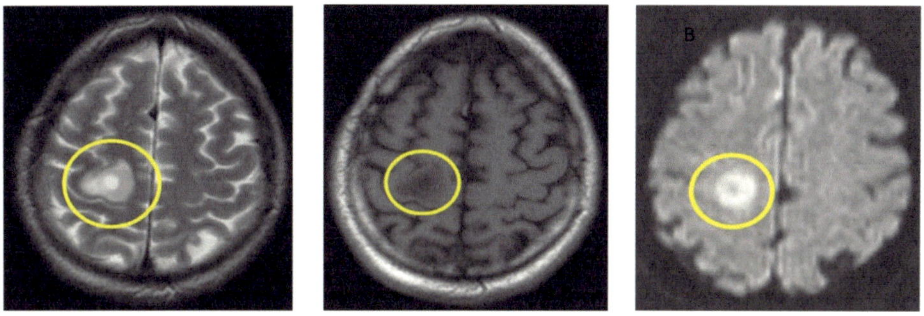

Figure 3.
MRI findings in a 55-year-old male with Baló's concentric sclerosis [37]. (A) Axial T2-weighted MRI reveals a well-defined, non-uniform lesion (circled) with alternating hyperintense and isointense bands corresponding to areas of demyelination and preserved myelin. Surrounding edema is present without significant mass effect. (Imaging parameters: 1.5 T magnet, 5 mm slice thickness, TR: 3300, TE: 97). (B) Axial T1-weighted MRI shows an irregular, round lesion (circled) with alternating hypointense and isointense bands, reflecting demyelinated and myelinated tissue. The lesion measures 1.9 cm × 1.6 cm × 1.1 cm in anteroposterior, transverse, and craniocaudal dimensions and is located in the right precentral gyrus, affecting the motor strip and hand region. Surrounding edema is present without mass effect. (Imaging parameters: 1.5 T magnet, 5 mm slice thickness, TR: 468, TE: 12). (C) Diffusion-weighted MRI (DWI) demonstrates a lesion (circled) with a low-signal central core and alternating high-signal intensity in the intermediate and outer rings. Active demyelination areas show restricted diffusion (high-signal intensity), while regions with facilitated diffusion appear as low-signal intensity. (Imaging parameters: 1.5 T magnet, 5 mm slice thickness, TR: 3600, TE: 89).

acute demyelination progresses concentrically from the center of the lesion. DWI typically visualizes fewer rings than T2-weighted imaging due to its lower spatial resolution [40–42].

The characteristic concentric ring pattern observed in MRI corresponds closely with histopathological findings in postmortem examinations (**Figure 4**) and is crucial in differentiating BCS from other CNS pathologies. These pathological features are often difficult to appreciate in biopsies due to the typically small sample sizes, which may not capture the full lesion architecture [37].

The differential diagnosis of BCS includes a range of demyelinating and neoplastic conditions. Among the primary considerations are ADEM, classic MS, and primary brain neoplasms such as gliomas [31]. Due to its radiological appearance, BCS can initially be mistaken for a high-grade glioma, particularly in cases where contrast-enhancing lesions are detected. High-grade gliomas on MRI typically present as enhancing masses surrounded by abnormal signal intensities—hypo- or iso-intense on T1-weighted images and hyperintense on T2-weighted and fluid-attenuated inversion recovery (FLAIR) sequences. The surrounding abnormality in gliomas, often referred to as "edema," may actually represent infiltrative tumor growth, whereas in metastatic tumors, it is more indicative of vasogenic edema without direct tumor invasion [43].

MRI remains superior to CT in distinguishing demyelinating diseases, including BCS, MS, and ADEM. Both MS and ADEM can closely resemble BCS on MRI; however, serial imaging can help differentiate them, as MS typically presents with new lesions over time, whereas BCS lesions may shrink or disappear on follow-up scans [16, 31, 44].

CT and CSF analysis can provide supplementary diagnostic insights alongside MRI. CT is generally not the primary imaging modality for diagnosing conditions such as ADEM, MS and BCS but remains a valuable tool for ruling out alternative diagnoses such as tumors, hemorrhages, or acute ischemic events [44]. CSF analysis plays a crucial role in distinguishing BCS from other demyelinating diseases. In BCS, CSF studies

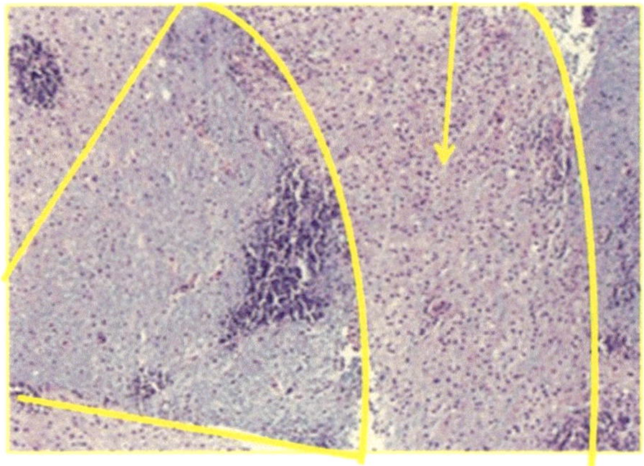

Figure 4.
Histopathological Findings in a 55-Year-Old Male with Baló's Concentric Sclerosis. The Luxol Fast Blue/H&E stain of the biopsy specimen highlights a hypercellular demyelinated lesion (pink, arrow) surrounded by relatively less cellular, preserved myelinated white matter (blue, outlined by yellow lines). Numerous histiocytes contain Luxol Fast Blue-positive myelin debris, indicative of active demyelination. Gliosis is present both within the demyelinated areas and in adjacent regions of intact myelin, reflecting the ongoing inflammatory process [37].

often reveal a mononuclear inflammatory response, with occasional oligoclonal bands. This contrasts with classical MS, where oligoclonal bands are more frequently detected at a significantly higher rate. Similarly, CSF findings in ADEM typically indicate pleocytosis and elevated protein levels, further differentiating ADEM from BCS [31]. A detailed investigation of BCS has underscored the critical role of oligodendrocyte pathology [45]. The morphological characteristics of BCS closely resemble the immunopathological pattern III described by Lucchinetti et al., which is associated with oligodendrocyte apoptosis and dysregulation of myelin proteins [46]. When lesion progression becomes more aggressive, oxidative tissue damage extends beyond the initially protected myelin rings, leading to new cycles of demyelination and remyelination, ultimately resulting in the characteristic concentric pattern seen in BCS [35]. CSF analysis in BCS is typically normal compared to classical MS, where intrathecal oligoclonal bands are detected in up to 98% of cases. In contrast, oligoclonal bands in BCS are found in only 35% of patients, suggesting a distinct immunopathogenic mechanism between the two diseases and reinforcing the concept that BCS represents a separate clinical entity rather than merely a variant of MS [1].

Patients with BCS may respond differently to immunosuppressive therapies compared to those with MS. The use of high-dose corticosteroids has been the primary treatment approach, with plasma exchange and immunosuppressive agents reserved for refractory cases [32]. Patients diagnosed early based on characteristic MRI findings have shown a favorable response to short-term, high-dose corticosteroid therapy, emphasizing the need for prompt imaging and clinical assessment [31]. Tissue biopsy is not routinely recommended for diagnosing BCS [31]. Instead, clinical-radiological correlation remains the cornerstone of diagnosis, helping to avoid unnecessary invasive procedures.

1.5 Myelinoclastic diffuse sclerosis or Schilder's disease

Myelinoclastic diffuse sclerosis (MDS), more commonly known as Schilder's disease, is a rare inflammatory DD of the CNS that was first described in 1912 by

Austrian psychiatrist Paul Ferdinand Schilder [47]. Unlike classical MS, where demyelination occurs in discrete plaques, MDS is characterized by widespread and confluent demyelination that is not confined to focal areas. This diffuse pattern differentiates it from MS and suggests a separate pathogenic mechanism. Subsequent studies have linked several cases of Schilder's diffuse sclerosis to defined metabolic disorders, particularly adrenoleukodystrophy. This association underscores the importance of metabolic screening in patients presenting with extensive demyelination, as misdiagnosing a metabolic disorder as a demyelinating disease could lead to inappropriate treatment strategies [48]. Historically, Schilder's disease has been a broad term encompassing various demyelinating conditions. Until 1985, it was used to describe multiple DDs with different etiologies, including adrenoleukodystrophy and subacute sclerosing panencephalitis. However, advances in neuropathology and neuroimaging have led to a refined understanding of these conditions, allowing for more precise classifications [49]. While MDS was initially thought to be a subtype of MS, more recent findings have demonstrated significant differences in clinical presentation, radiological features, laboratory markers, and pathological findings that distinguish it from other demyelinating diseases (**Table 1**) [50].

MDS is a rare DD primarily affecting children and young adults. Poser [51, 52] proposed a practical definition for its diagnosis, which includes the following criteria: (1) a subacute or chronic DD presenting with one or two bilaterally symmetrical white matter lesions measuring at least 2 × 3 cm in two dimensions, (**Figure 5**), (2) primary involvement of the centrum semiovale, (3) absence of additional demyelinating lesions based on clinical, paraclinical, or imaging findings, and (4) exclusion of adrenoleukodystrophy as a differential diagnosis.

In 1986, Poser proposed diagnostic criteria for the non-invasive identification of Schilder's disease, distinguishing it from early MS based on several key clinical and laboratory features. These criteria included atypical symptoms for early MS, normal or non-specific CSF findings, extensive bilateral demyelination in the cerebral white matter, absence of fever, lack of preceding viral or mycoplasma infection, and normal serum levels of very long-chain fatty acids [54].

Histopathologically, Schilder's disease exhibits widespread inflammatory demyelination similar to MS, though with significantly larger and more diffuse areas of demyelination, leading to its classification as "myelinoclastic diffuse sclerosis" (**Figure 6**).

The exact relationship between Schilder's disease and MS remains uncertain. Poser suggested that Schilder's disease may represent a transitional condition between Schilder's disease and classical MS. The primary distinctions include a more aggressive clinical progression, the absence of CSF pleocytosis, and a lack of oligoclonal bands, which are typically observed in MS [50].

The etiology of Schilder's disease remains unknown, with its symptoms attributed to widespread demyelination throughout the CNS, leading to impaired neural transmission and progressively worsening neurological decline. Clinical manifestations vary and may include cognitive and psychiatric disturbances, aphasia, ataxia, dementia, hemiplegia, increased intracranial pressure, cortical blindness, deafness, tremors, seizures, attention deficits, headaches, muscle weakness, vomiting, visual impairment, personality changes, and balance difficulties [55]. The disease course is highly variable; some patients experience a relentless progression leading to death, while others undergo remissions interspersed with exacerbations. Each relapse tends to be more severe than the previous, and remissions become increasingly incomplete over time, eventually leading to fatal outcomes [56, 57].

	MS	ADEM	Schilder's disease	Devic's syndrome
Age	>10 years	<10 years	5–14 years	20–40 years
Gender	M > F	M = F	M = F	F > M
Prior flu	Variable	Very frequent	–	Frequent
Encephalopathy	rare	required	–	–
Course	RR, SP, PP, PR	Relapsing/monophasic/ multiphasic	Monophasic-not remitting/remitting/ progressive	Monophasic/ relapsing
Topography	Optic nerve cerebellum brainstem central white matter	Subcortical brainstem thalamus	Centrum semiovale parieto-occipital white matter	Optic nerve/spinal cord
Relapses	Slight to moderate	Moderate	Severe	Severe
Brain MRI	Small lesions	Large, symmetric lesions	Large lesions	Non-specific
Spinal cord	<1 segment,	–	–	>3 segment,
MRI	Marginal			Central
CSF cells	<50 lymphocytes	>50 lymphocytes	Normal	>50 PMN
CSF oligoclonal bands	Positive	Variable	Negative	Negative
NMO-IgG	<10%	–	–	>70%

Table 1.
Comparative clinical, CSF, and MRI features of multiple sclerosis (MS), acute disseminated encephalomyelitis (ADEM), Schilder's disease, and Devic's syndrome [50].

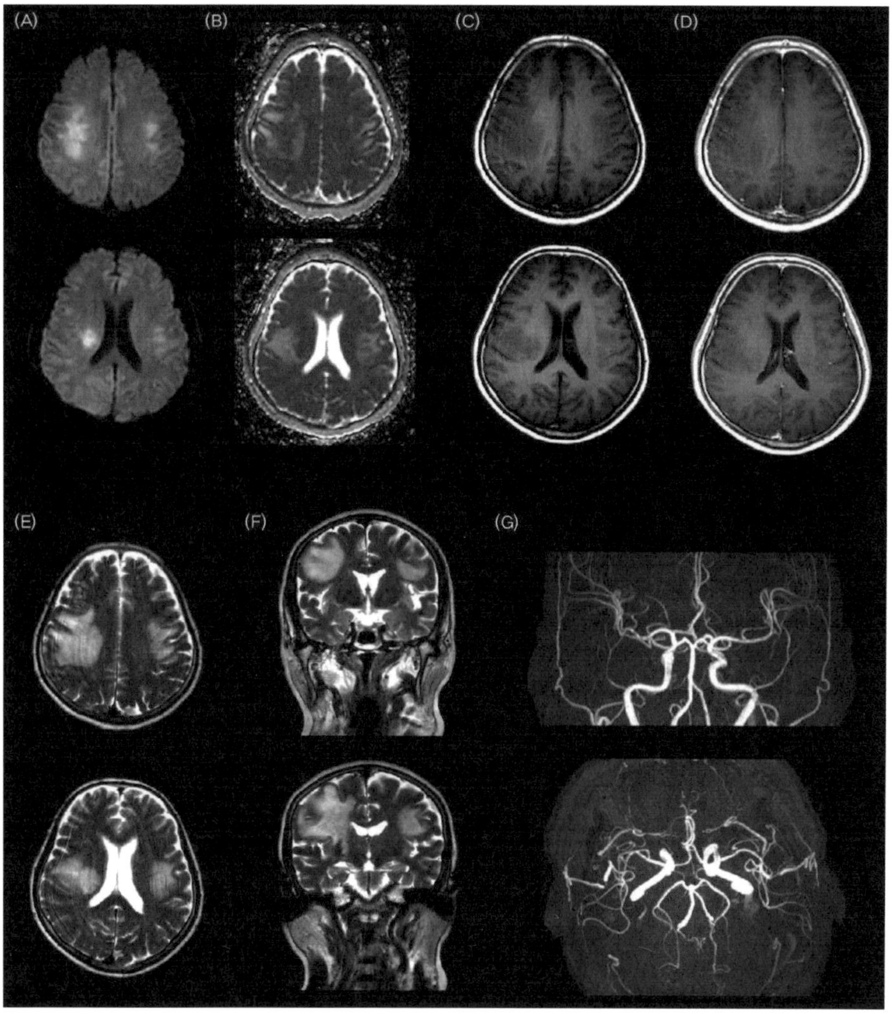

Figure 5.
MRI and MRA findings in a pathology-confirmed case of Schilder's disease [53]. (A) Diffusion-weighted imaging, (B) apparent diffusion coefficient, (C) T1 weighted, (D) gadolinium enhanced T1 weighted, (E) axial T2-weighted, and (F) coronal T2-weighted MRI scans taken on the ninth day post-onset. (G) Magnetic resonance angiography (MRA) obtained on the third day post-onset. The MRI reveals bilateral, sharply demarcated plaque-like demyelinating lesions in (A), (E), and (F). Partial high-signal intensities are visible in (B), while (C) and (D) show low-signal intensities without gadolinium enhancement. The MRA (G) demonstrates normal vascular structures.

Schilder's disease has historically been regarded as a uniformly fatal disorder [57, 58]. However, its prognosis is highly variable, following one of three potential courses: a monophasic non-remitting form, a relapsing-remitting pattern, or a progressive form characterized by accumulating deficits.

The differentiation of Schilder's disease from other conditions, such as brain tumors or abscesses, is a significant diagnostic challenge. Due to the large size and appearance of demyelinating lesions, imaging alone is often insufficient for definitive diagnosis, and invasive procedures like brain biopsy remain the gold standard [54].

The therapeutic approach to Schilder's disease aligns with standard MS treatments. Management strategies primarily involve high-dose corticosteroids,

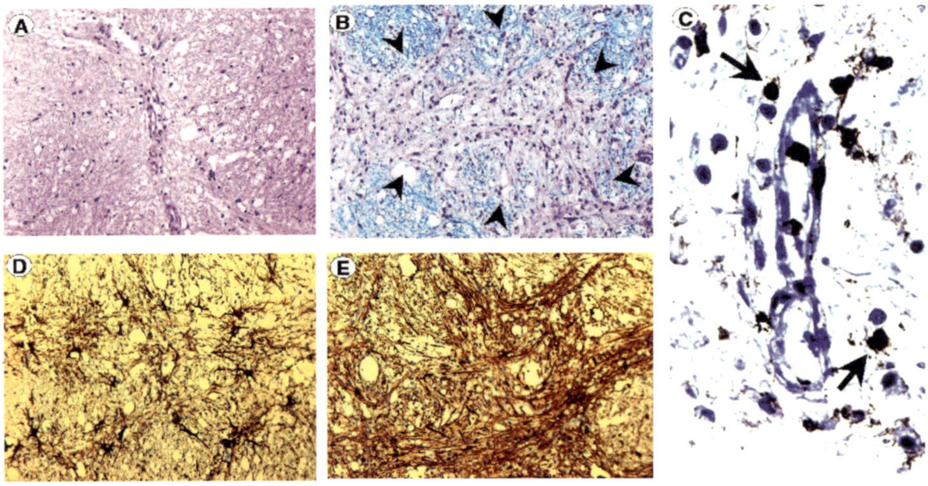

Figure 6.
Histopathological findings in a pathology-confirmed case of Schilder's disease [53]. **(A)** *Hematoxylin and eosin (H&E) staining shows perivascular infiltrates composed of a few lymphocytes and macrophages (×200). (B) Luxol fast blue staining highlights an area of demyelination (arrowheads) with a lighter blue hue (×200). (C) CD45 immunohistochemistry reveals immunoreactive lymphocytes (arrows) within the perivascular space (×400). (D) Glial fibrillary acidic protein (GFAP) staining demonstrates reactive astrocytes in the demyelinated lesions (×200). (E) Neurofilament staining indicates well-preserved neuropils within the affected regions (×200).*

immunosuppressive agents, and symptomatic therapy. Immunoglobulin therapy has been attempted with inconsistent results—demonstrating limited efficacy in some cases while proving ineffective in others [57, 59]. Additional immunosuppressive therapies, such as cyclophosphamide followed by azathioprine, have shown variable outcomes [59].

1.6 Neuromyelitis optica or Devic's syndrome

1.6.1 Introduction

Devic's disease, also known as neuromyelitis optica (NMO), is an idiopathic inflammatory DD of the CNS that primarily affects the optic nerves and spinal cord. The condition is marked by recurrent episodes of optic neuritis and myelitis, often leading to severe visual impairment and motor disability. The earliest known description of a patient suffering from visual loss and spinal cord dysfunction dates back to the nineteenth century, with contributions from various researchers, including Antoine Portal. Other significant early observations were made by Pescetto, Durrant, Lockhard, and Clarke [60]. The association between optic neuritis and spinal cord disease was first formally acknowledged by Allbutt in 1870, while Erb provided the first comprehensive description of NMO in 1880 [61]. In 1894, the French neurologist Eugène Devic, alongside his student Fernand Gault, introduced the term "neuromyelitis optica" and described a clinical syndrome consisting of optic neuritis and acute transverse myelitis as its key features [60–62]. Initially, NMO was thought to follow a monophasic course, but subsequent case reports—including those by Beck in 1927 and McAlpine in 1938—identified patients who experienced a relapsing-remitting disease pattern, further complicating the classification of the disorder [61]. A major breakthrough in understanding NMO came in 2004 when Lennon and Wingerchuk discovered NMO immunoglobulin G (NMO-IgG), a specific autoantibody that distinguished NMO from MS [63]. In a subsequent breakthrough the following year, Lennon and colleagues identified AQP4 as the target antigen for NMO-IgG. AQP4 primarily expressed on astrocyte foot processes within the CNS, plays a key role in blood-brain barrier integrity [64]. The detection of anti-AQP4 antibodies in the serum of NMO patients has since become a defining biomarker of the disease.

1.6.2 Diagnostic criteria for NMO and NMO spectrum disorders

In 2006, Wingerchuk and colleagues [65] revised the diagnostic criteria for NMO, which became widely accepted for several years. Advancements in the understanding of NMO's immunopathogenesis, along with the identification of varying clinical and radiological presentations, led to the realization that NMO represents a broader disease spectrum. As a result, the term "neuromyelitis optica spectrum disorders" (NMOSD) was introduced to encompass AQP4-IgG-positive NMO cases and other limited forms of the disease [62, 66].

In 2015, the International Panel for NMO Diagnosis (IPND) established an updated "International Consensus Diagnostic Criteria for NMOSD" [67]. Under these new guidelines, NMOSD is classified based on serologic status into NMOSD with or without AQP4-IgG (**Figure 7**). For NMOSD without AQP4-IgG, stricter diagnostic requirements apply compared to previous classifications.

1.6.3 Clinical features and laboratory findings of NMO

NMO predominantly affects women more frequently than men, with female-to-male ratios ranging from 2:1 to as high as 10:1 in reported studies [62, 66]. It is estimated that approximately 90% of individuals with relapsing NMO are female. The median age of disease onset is around 39 years, although cases have been reported in both pediatric and elderly populations [62]. NMO has a global prevalence of approximately one to three per 100,000 individuals [66]. The frequency of NMO cases varies across different ethnic populations; while it remains relatively rare in Caucasian populations (1–2% of MS cases), it is significantly more prevalent in regions such as the West Indies and Asia, where NMO constitutes 20–48% of DDs [62, 68]. Although NMO is typically sporadic, familial cases have been reported, accounting for approximately 3% of cases [66, 68, 69]. Genetic studies suggest that certain human leukocyte antigen (HLA) alleles, including DRB1*0301* in white populations and *DPB1*0501 in Asians, may be associated with an increased risk of developing NMO [62, 70].

Certain external factors, such as pregnancy and the postpartum period, have been linked to the onset or relapse of NMO [66, 68].

Clinically, NMO may present as either a monophasic or a relapsing disorder, with 80–90% of patients experiencing recurrent relapses. The hallmark features of NMO include optic neuritis, characterized by ocular pain and vision impairment, and acute transverse myelitis, which presents with motor dysfunction, sensory deficits, and bladder dysfunction. Additional neurological symptoms include Lhermitte's sign, paroxysmal tonic spasms, radicular pain, and in cases of cervical myelitis extending to the brainstem, nausea, hiccups, and respiratory failure. Less common manifestations include endocrinopathies, encephalopathy, coma, cerebral syndromes, and posterior reversible encephalopathy syndrome (PRES) [66].

Following the initial disease attack, 60% of patients experience a second relapse within 1 year, with 90% relapsing within 3 years. Patients who test

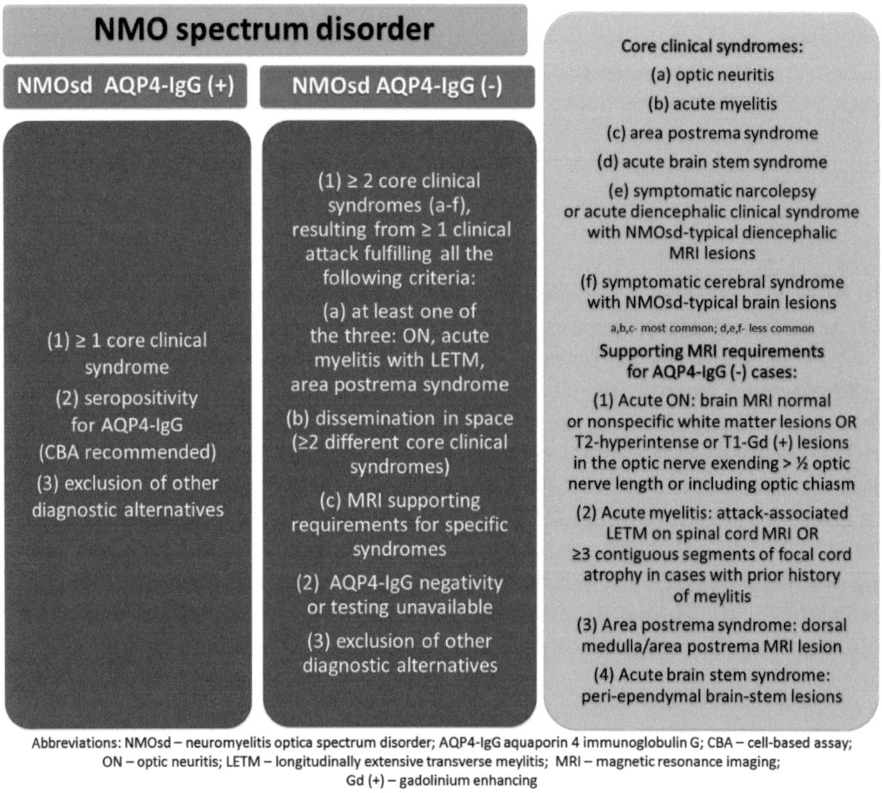

Figure 7.
Diagnostic criteria for neuromyelitis spectrum according to International Panel for Neuromyelitis Optica (NMO) Diagnosis (2015) [67]. This figure outlines the diagnostic framework for NMOSD, incorporating clinical and serological criteria. Key components include the presence of core clinical syndromes, AQP4-IgG serostatus, and characteristic MRI findings.

positive for AQP4-IgG and present with recurrent ON or the first episode of longitudinally extensive transverse myelitis (LETM) face an elevated risk of subsequent relapses. Unlike MS, NMO relapses tend to be more severe, leading to progressive neurological impairment. Within 5 years, over 50% of relapsing patients experience significant disability, such as unilateral or bilateral blindness, or require ambulatory assistance [62]. The proportion of patients with persistent monoplegia or paraplegia is notably higher in relapsing cases (52%) compared to monophasic cases (31%), and respiratory failure occurs more frequently in relapsing NMO (33% vs. 9%) [61].

The prognosis of relapsing NMO is generally poorer than that of MS, with factors such as frequent early relapses, severe initial attacks, and coexistence of systemic autoimmune diseases (e.g., systemic lupus erythematosus) indicating worse outcomes [62]. The five-year survival rate is approximately 90% for monophasic patients and 68% for relapsing cases, with respiratory failure being a primary cause of death in severe cases [61].

Diagnostic imaging plays a crucial role in differentiating NMO from MS. While the initial brain MRI is often normal, optic nerve gadolinium enhancement and brainstem lesions may be present. Spinal cord MRI commonly reveals longitudinal lesions extending over three or more vertebral segments, a hallmark finding with 98% sensitivity and 83% specificity for NMO (**Figure 8**) [65]. CSF analysis further assists in differential diagnosis, as significant pleocytosis and elevated protein levels are more common in NMO compared to MS, while oligoclonal IgG bands are rare (15–30%) in NMO patients [61, 62, 66]. The detection of AQP4-IgG remains the most specific biomarker for NMO, aiding both diagnosis and prognosis [62–64, 68]. These autoantibodies demonstrate a sensitivity of approximately 73% and a specificity of 91% for clinically confirmed NMO cases [62, 63]. Notably, a subset of patients with NMO, estimated at 10–25%, are seronegative for AQP4-IgG [62]. In AQP4-IgG seronegative patients, alternative autoantibodies have been identified, including aquaporin-1 antibodies (AQP1-Abs) [70] and myelin oligodendrocyte glycoprotein antibodies (MOG-IgGs) [72].

1.6.4 Immunopathogenesis of NMO

The precise etiology of NMO remains unknown, though numerous infectious and autoimmune triggers have been implicated. Various antecedent or concurrent infections, including tuberculosis and viral infections, as well as vaccinations and systemic autoimmune disorders such as systemic lupus erythematosus (SLE), rheumatoid arthritis, Sjögren's syndrome, and Hashimoto's thyroiditis, have been associated with the onset or relapse of NMO [62, 73].

Compared to classical MS, NMO is distinguished by more extensive complement activation, a higher degree of eosinophilic infiltration, and greater vascular damage, reinforcing its classification as an antibody-mediated disorder. This suggests that NMO pathogenesis is primarily driven by a Th2-polarized immune

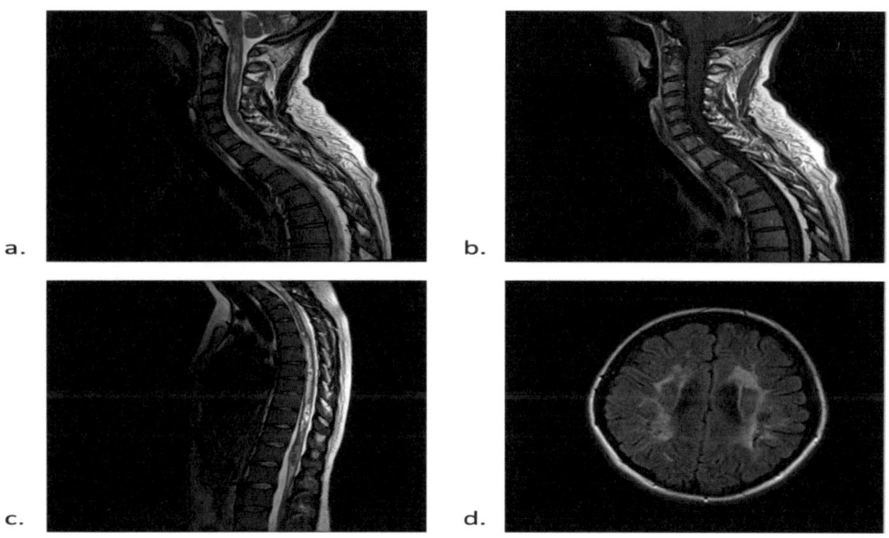

Figure 8.
Neuroradiological findings in Neuromyelitis Optica Spectrum Disorder (NMOSD) [71]. MRI scans of a 51-year-old female with AQP4-IgG (+) NMOSD showing a longitudinally extensive T2-hyperintense lesion in the cervical spinal cord extending into the brainstem (a) and corresponding T1-hypointensities indicative of focal spinal cord atrophy (b). MRI scans of a 20-year-old female with AQP4-IgG (+) NMOSD, demonstrating nearly complete longitudinal involvement of the thoracic spinal cord (c), and brain FLAIR images with lesions that do not meet MS diagnostic criteria (d) [71].

response [74, 75]. The presence of a pathogenic autoantibody, termed NMO-IgG in patient serum is now recognized as a highly specific biomarker that distinguishes NMO from MS and other inflammatory CNS disorders [64, 73]. The circulating NMO-IgG gains access to its target, AQP4, through breaches in the blood-brain barrier. The binding of AQP4-IgG to astrocytes leads to complement activation, culminating in astrocyte destruction, secondary neuronal damage, and subsequent demyelination (**Figure 9**).

1.6.5 Treatment strategies of NMO

The treatment of NMO involves both acute attack management and long-term relapse prevention. During acute episodes, hospitalization is often required, particularly in cases involving ventilatory failure [77].

The first-line therapy for acute attacks includes high-dose intravenous methylprednisolone, administered over a five-day course (30 mg/kg/day for patients under 30 kg and up to 1 g/day for those over 30 kg) [77, 78]. In cases where corticosteroids fail to produce an adequate response, plasma exchange (55 ml/kg every other day) or intravenous immunoglobulin (IVIg) therapy (0.4 g/kg/day for 5 days) may be employed. These therapies have shown particular efficacy in pediatric patients [78, 79].

For relapse prevention, long-term immunosuppressive therapy plays a crucial role. A study involving seven patients demonstrated that a maintenance regimen combining azathioprine (2.5–3 mg/kg/day) with prednisone (1 mg/kg/day) effectively prevented relapses. Over time, prednisone was tapered gradually once azathioprine reached full therapeutic efficacy (typically after 4–6 months). After 2 months, prednisone was reduced to a maintenance dose of 10 mg/day, resulting in no recorded relapses and improved functional outcomes during follow-up [77].

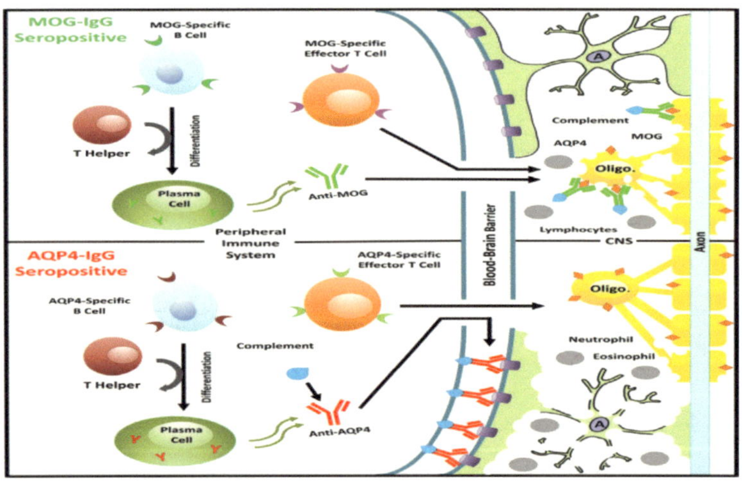

Figure 9.
Mechanisms of AQP4- and MOG-specific antibody-mediated CNS damage [76]. The upper panel illustrates how MOG-specific effector T-cells initiate CNS inflammation, leading to lymphocyte accumulation. Once inside the CNS, MOG-specific IgG binds to myelin and myelin-forming oligodendrocytes, promoting demyelination and oligodendrocyte damage. The lower panel depicts the role of AQP4-specific IgG, which is produced by plasma cells with the assistance of antigen-specific T-helper cells. CNS inflammation in AQP4-mediated disease is characterized by neutrophil and eosinophil infiltration. AQP4-IgG1 binds to AQP4 water channels on astrocyte end-feet, leading to complement activation and astrocyte injury.

Other immunosuppressive agents, including mycophenolate mofetil, rituximab, mitoxantrone, and cyclophosphamide, have also demonstrated effectiveness in inducing disease remission in patients unresponsive to initial treatments [62, 80–82].

Recent advances in NMO research have led to the development of novel therapies specifically targeting the immunopathogenic mechanisms underlying the disease [60]. Such therapies are aquaporumab [83], sivelestat [84], eculizumab [85], and tocilizumab [86].

1.7 Marburg's acute MS

Marburg's variant of MS is an aggressive, monophasic form of the disease characterized by a rapid and severe clinical progression, often leading to death within 1–6 months from symptom onset or resulting in severe disability. This fulminant variant was first described in 1906 by Otto Marburg, who documented three cases of MS with extensive CNS lesions and rapid deterioration [34]. Since its identification, this severe form has been referred to as Marburg's variant of MS. Patients typically present with focal neurological deficits, seizures, or rapid neurological decline, often culminating in death within weeks to months due to brainstem involvement [87, 88].

Pathologically, Marburg's MS is distinguished by highly destructive lesions with significant macrophage infiltration, acute axonal injury, and necrosis (**Figure 10**) [90]. Compared to classical MS, the lesions in Marburg's variant exhibit extreme tissue destruction. Inflammatory demyelination may also extend to the peripheral nervous system, rather than being confined solely to the CNS [48]. Despite some similarities in lesion distribution to chronic MS, Marburg's variant is distinguished by its uniform and widespread demyelination. The plaques exhibit consistency across affected regions, aligning with the disease's monophasic nature. However, even within acute MS, temporal dissemination may occur, leading to variations in lesion progression [91].

Clinically, Marburg's variant differs from classical MS due to its rapid disease course and severe presentation, with patients experiencing profound neurological deterioration within a short timeframe. Death is most commonly attributed to brainstem involvement. The precise mechanisms responsible for the extreme disease severity remain unclear, with hypotheses suggesting an exceptionally aggressive immune-mediated attack or dominance of a specific immune effector mechanism. Radiologically, lesions exhibit substantial mass effect and edema, making them difficult to differentiate from tumefactive MS or ADEM. Marburg's variant is considered an extreme end of the demyelinating disease spectrum, and distinguishing it from other fulminant MS variants in clinical practice remains challenging.

Due to advances in anti-inflammatory therapies and intensive care, acute MS is now extremely rare. Severe forms such as Marburg's variant and Balo's concentric sclerosis account for less than 4% of all MS cases. The National MS Society estimates the prevalence of MS to be approximately 135 per 100,000 individuals in the United States, with a total MS population of around 400,000.

The clinical course of Marburg's variant is aggressive and frequently fatal. The underlying etiology of its malignant progression remains unclear, but it is hypothesized that the severity could be linked to immune-mediated destruction of vital areas such as the brainstem or an atypically aggressive immunopathological mechanism

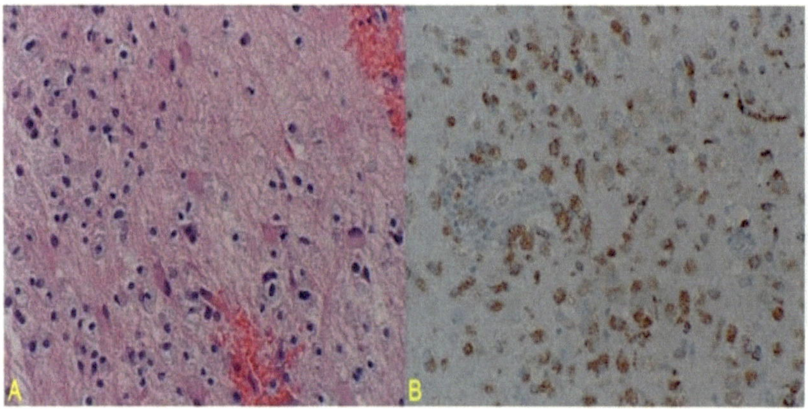

Figure 10.
pathologic features of white matter lesions [89]. (A) Hematoxylin & eosin (H&E) staining reveals white matter infiltration by macrophages and reactive astrocytes. (B) CD68 immunohistochemical staining highlights histiocytes localized within the white matter, with sparing of the gray matter.

[92]. Biochemical analyses suggest that myelin basic protein (MBP) isoforms in Marburg's variant differ from those in classical MS. Specifically, Marburg's MS is associated with an 18.5 kDa MBP isoform that is less cationic due to increased deamination of arginyl residues into citrulline [87, 93, 94]. This structural alteration reduces the stability of the central myelin sheath, contributing to the rapid demyelination and tissue destruction characteristic of the disease [95].

The clinical presentation of Marburg's MS is marked by acute neurological deficits, which may include decreased consciousness, hemiplegia, aphasia, and seizures, depending on lesion location. Symptoms evolve more rapidly than in conventional MS subtypes. Demyelinating plaques are often present in both supratentorial and infratentorial structures, with large tumor-like demyelinating lesions frequently affecting the centrum semiovale [92]. Brain and spinal cord MRI typically reveal extensive T2-weighted hyperintense lesions disseminated throughout the hemispheric white matter and brainstem, often associated with mass effect and edema (**Figure 11**). Gadolinium enhancement is often present, indicating active inflammation. MR spectroscopy findings include increased choline peaks and reduced N-acetyl-aspartate (NAA), consistent with axonal damage observed in other DDs.

CSF analysis in Marburg's MS generally shows elevated protein levels, with minimal or no pleocytosis. Oligoclonal bands, commonly observed in classical MS, are less frequently detected in Marburg's variant. Neuropathological examinations typically reveal acute plaques with extensive demyelination, though occasional chronic plaques have also been described. Other pathological features include severe oligodendrocyte loss, axonal preservation, infiltration of giant astrocytes, and pronounced macrophage and microglial activation. Reactive astrocytosis is also a prominent finding [92, 97].

Despite its rarity, Marburg's variant remains an important consideration in rapidly progressive DDs. Given its aggressive course and poor prognosis, early recognition and intervention are critical, though treatment options remain limited. The differential diagnosis of NMOSD includes a broad range of conditions, including multifocal

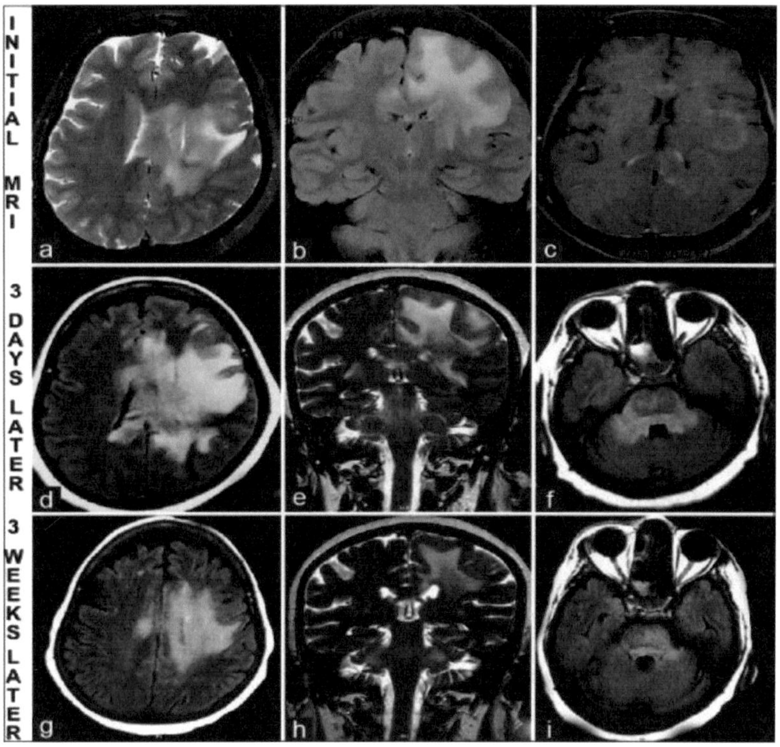

Figure 11.
MRI brain imaging across disease progression [96]. Initial presentation: (a) T2-weighted axial and (b) T2 FLAIR coronal images reveal a hyperintense lesion affecting the centrum semiovale, corpus callosum, deep cerebral nuclei, and corpus callosum. (c) T1-weighted contrast axial image shows ill-defined enhancement within the lesion. MRI 3 days later: (d) T2-weighted axial, (e) T2 FLAIR coronal, and (f) T2 FLAIR axial images demonstrate lesion enlargement with bilateral extension into the brainstem. MRI 3 weeks later: (g) T2 FLAIR, (h) T2-weighted coronal, and (i) T2 FLAIR axial images indicate lesion regression.

brain tumors, infectious, metabolic, vascular, and other DDs. Among the demyelinating diseases, BCS, Schilder's diffuse sclerosis, and ADEM are key considerations due to their overlapping clinical and radiological features [98–100].

The primary treatment for Marburg's MS is intravenous corticosteroids, but this approach is often insufficient in severe cases. Patients unresponsive to steroids may benefit from IVIg or cycles of plasmapheresis, which have demonstrated positive effects in refractory cases [101]. Mitoxantrone, a potent immunosuppressive and immunomodulatory anthracenedione, has shown efficacy in aggressive MS subtypes as well as in some cases of Marburg MS [88, 102]. Additionally, high-dose cyclophosphamide has shown promise in patients who failed first-line treatments [103].

1.8 Acute disseminated encephalomyelitis

1.8.1 Introduction

ADEM, also referred to as post-infectious encephalomyelitis, is a severe, monophasic, inflammatory autoimmune disorder affecting the CNS and spinal cord. It is distinct from MS in both pathology and clinical course. ADEM is frequently triggered by a systemic infection or, less commonly, by vaccination occurring 1–2 weeks before the initiation of neurological symptoms [104, 105]. Identifiable infections or immunizations have been reported in approximately 50–85% of cases [106, 107].

ADEM predominantly affects the pediatric population, where MS is less common. Its incidence is estimated at 0.4–0.8 per 100,000 individuals per year, with the highest prevalence in children under 10 years of age [104, 108, 109]. The higher incidence in children is thought to be related to immature myelin, a relatively underdeveloped immune response, and the increased frequency of viral infections in childhood compared to adulthood [110].

The disease is observed more frequently in males than females, with an estimated male-to-female ratio of approximately 1.3–1. The condition also exhibits seasonal patterns, with a higher incidence during winter and spring. Several factors influence the risk of developing ADEM, including genetic susceptibility, prior exposure to infectious agents, immunization history, and lighter skin pigmentation.

Diagnosis of ADEM is primarily based on clinical assessment, supplemented by characteristic findings on neuroimaging [111].

1.8.2 Pathophysiology of ADEM

The exact pathophysiological mechanisms of ADEM are not yet fully elucidated. However, it is believed to result from an autoimmune reaction triggered by environmental stimuli such as infections (influenza virus, hepatitis A, cytomegalovirus, Epstein-Barr virus, herpes simplex virus, human herpesvirus-6, human immunodeficiency virus (HIV), beta-hemolytic Streptococcus, Borrelia burgdorferi and Leptospira) [112–114] or vaccinations (for rabies, measles, pertussis, tetanus, influenza, hepatitis B, diphtheria, rubella, pneumococcus, varicella, smallpox, human papillomavirus (HPV), and poliomyelitis) in genetically susceptible individuals.

Historically, before the implementation of immunization programs, ADEM was most frequently associated with measles, rubella, mumps, varicella, and smallpox. In contemporary settings, ADEM is more commonly triggered by gastrointestinal or respiratory viral infections [115, 116].

The incidence of post-vaccination ADEM has declined in recent years, likely due to advancements in vaccine formulation and production techniques [117].

Proposed mechanisms for ADEM are:

1. Molecular mimicry, wherein pathogens or vaccines share antigenic epitopes with host CNS myelin antigens, triggering an immune response against myelin-reactive T cells [118].

2. Direct CNS infection which subsequently triggers a secondary inflammatory cascade which compromises the integrity of the blood-brain barrier, allowing CNS-specific antigens to enter the peripheral circulation, where they are recognized and processed by the immune system. This process may lead to an autoimmune response targeting the CNS [118].

3. The role of autoantibodies: Elevated anti-MBP antibody titers have been observed in patients with postvaccinal ADEM, particularly in cases linked to

the Semple rabies vaccine. Antibasal ganglia antibodies have been detected in cases of post-streptococcal ADEM [119]. Additionally, elevated serum anti-MOG antibody titers have been reported in 20–47% of pediatric patients with acute CNS demyelination, with the highest levels seen in ADEM. These antibodies in ADEM tend to decline over time, whereas they persist in MS patients, providing a potential distinguishing biomarker between the two conditions [120–122].

4. Cytokines and chemokines: CSF studies indicate a Th2-skewed immune response, elevated levels of chemokines such as CCL17 and CCL22, which are associated with macrophage and microglial activation, of eosinophil- and neutrophil-associated chemokines, of proinflammatory cytokines, including interleukin (IL)-6 and tumor necrosis factor-alpha (TNF-α), as well as the anti-inflammatory cytokine IL-10, in ADEM [123, 124].

5. Genetic predisposition: Several studies have identified associations with major histocompatibility complex (MHC) class II alleles, including HLA-DRB1*1501 and HLA-DRB5*0101 in Korean populations, as well as HLA-DRB3*0202 and HLA-DQB1*0502 in cases of acute necrotizing encephalopathy. Russian studies have reported associations with HLA-DRB1*01 and HLA-DRB*03(017) [118].

1.8.3 Clinical features of ADEM

1.8.3.1 Clinical presentation of ADEM

ADEM often presents with a range of non-specific constitutional symptoms, including fever, headache, fatigue, malaise, nausea, and vomiting. According to the International Pediatric MS Study Group (IPMSSG) criteria, a definitive ADEM diagnosis requires both encephalopathy and polyfocal neurological deficits [107]. Encephalopathy, in this context, refers to altered mental status, which may manifest as irritability, confusion, psychosis, somnolence, or even coma. Polyfocal neurological deficits encompass motor and sensory impairments such as paraparesis and tetraparesis, along with potential brainstem dysfunction, which can cause dysarthria, oculomotor disturbances, or other neurological symptoms like seizures, meningismus, ataxia, aphasia, nystagmus, optic neuritis, urinary retention, elevated intracranial pressure, and extrapyramidal signs.

Typically, ADEM follows a monophasic disease course, with a single demyelinating episode. The severity of symptoms often fluctuates within the first 3 months. If a second inflammatory demyelinating event occurs beyond this period, the condition is classified as multiphasic ADEM. The disease progression is generally rapid, with the most severe deficits emerging within a few days of onset (mean time to peak symptom severity is approximately 4.5 days) [125].

In younger children, particularly those under 5 years of age, ADEM can present with cerebellar mutism and prolonged focal motor seizures [108, 115, 116, 125]. Additionally, a distinct form of ADEM has been linked to group A beta-hemolytic streptococcal infections, characterized by significant behavioral disturbances, dystonic movements, and basal ganglia abnormalities on MRI, in addition to the characteristic white matter lesions [120].

The diagnostic criteria (**Table 2**) established by International Pediatric MS Study Group (IPMSSG) are primarily designed for pediatric cases of ADEM, whereas no universally accepted guidelines exist for diagnosing the condition in adults. Research suggests that ADEM in adults is associated with a poorer prognosis compared to pediatric cases [127, 128].

1.8.3.2 Neuroimaging pattern of ADEM

MRI is the preferred imaging modality for ADEM, revealing hyperintense, heterogeneous, and poorly marginated lesions on T2-weighted, fluid-attenuated inversion recovery (FLAIR), proton density, and echo-planar diffusion sequences (**Figure 12**). These lesions are not typically seen on T1-weighted sequences unless they are particularly large, in which case they may appear hypointense. Imaging

ADEM	Single polyfocal clinical CNS event with presumed inflammatory cause
	Encephalopathy that cannot be explained by fever
	MRI typically shows diffuse, poorly demarcated, large >1-2 cm lesions predominantly involving cerebral white matter; T1 hypointense white matter lesions are rare; deep gray matter lesions (e.g., thalamus or basal ganglia) can be present
	No new symptoms, signs, or MRI findings after 3 months of initial ADEM
Multiphasic ADEM	New event of ADEM 3 months or more after initial event that can be associated with new or re-emergence of prior clinical and MRI findings
ADEM-ON	At least one subsequent attack of optic neuritis, without encephalopathy, at least 3 months after initial ADEM
ADEM-MS	ADEM followed 3 months later by a non-encephalopathic clinical event with new lesions on brain MRI consistent with MS
ADEM-NMOSD	ADEM followed 3 months later by ON, myelitis, or area postrema syndrome, fulfilling NMOSD diagnostic criteria

Table 2.
Criteria for ADEM and relapsing disorders following ADEM [126].

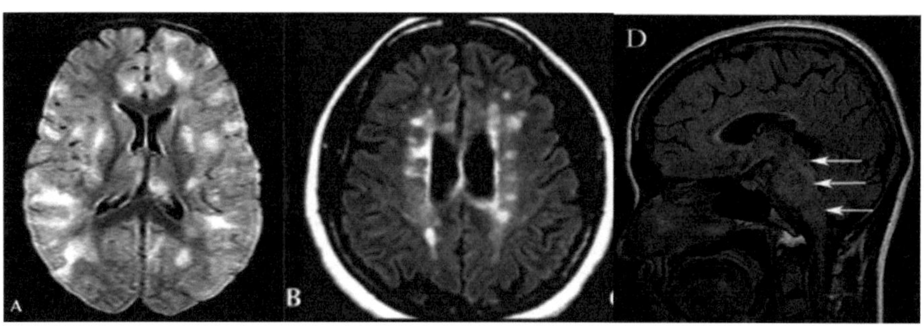

Figure 12.
Neuroimaging Features of ADEM and MS (A) Axial FLAIR MRI demonstrating bilateral, globular hyperintense lesions in the cortical gray matter, centrum semiovale, and deep gray nuclei, characteristic of ADEM. (B) Axial FLAIR MRI showing ovoid, periventricular hyperintensities, typical of MS plaques [129]. (C) Sagittal FLAIR MRI revealing multiple, poorly demarcated lesions in the midbrain, pons, and medulla, consistent with ADEM [130].

may show a solitary lesion or multiple, widespread asymmetric lesions distributed across both white (e.g., periventricular and subcortical) and gray matter (e.g., basal ganglia, thalamus, and cortex) structures [131–133]. ADEM most commonly presents with multiple, bilateral lesions, but infratentorial involvement in the brainstem, cerebellum, and spinal cord may also be observed. In pediatric cases, lesions frequently involve deep gray matter, whereas in adults, periventricular lesions are more common [125].

A key distinguishing feature of ADEM lesions on MRI is their poorly defined borders, in contrast to the sharply demarcated lesions characteristic of MS. Additional MRI findings favoring an MS diagnosis over ADEM include the presence of two or more periventricular lesions, T1 black holes, and an absence of a bilateral lesion distribution at the initial demyelinating event [134]. Although MRI is the imaging gold standard, CT scans may be used in urgent settings to exclude alternative diagnoses. The prevalence of gadolinium-enhancing lesions on T1-weighted MRI in ADEM varies widely (8–100%), depend on the inflammatory stage at the time of imaging. Unlike MS, ADEM lesions generally appear at a uniform stage of development.

MRI findings in ADEM can evolve over time. Delayed lesion development has been reported in both pediatric and adult cases. Five proposed MRI subtypes of ADEM in children include [125, 135]:

1. ADEM with small lesions (<5 mm)

2. ADEM with large, confluent, or tumefactive lesions, often with mass effect

3. ADEM with symmetrical bithalamic involvement

4. Acute hemorrhagic encephalomyelitis (AHEM) characterized by hemorrhagic lesions

5. ADEM with a pseudo-leukodystrophic pattern, presenting as diffuse, symmetrical white matter involvement [100].

Serial MRI studies play a key role in confirming ADEM. The development of new lesions over time is uncommon in ADEM but serves as a key indicator for MS diagnosis [136].

1.8.3.3 Other laboratory features of ADEM

1.8.3.3.1 Cerebrospinal fluid

CSF analysis is often normal but may exhibit abnormalities in 50–80% of ADEM cases. Common findings include increased pressure, lymphocytic pleocytosis (up to 1000 cells/mm^3, sometimes with an initial polymorphonuclear predominance), and elevated protein levels (typically <1.0 mg/L). CSF may also show elevated gamma globulin, IgG, and myelin basic protein, indicative of CNS demyelination. Glucose levels are typically normal. Oligoclonal bands are rare in ADEM but, when present, tend to diminish as the disease resolves [137].

1.8.3.3.2 Electroencephalography

EEG abnormalities are frequently observed in ADEM but lack specificity. Findings range from mild generalized slowing to severe abnormalities, including focal slowing and epileptiform discharges. In some cases, EEG findings correlate with disease severity. EEG can be particularly useful in distinguishing ADEM from psychiatric disorders [138].

1.8.3.3.3 Pathologic findings in ADEM

The hallmark lesions of ADEM predominantly involve small veins encircled by foamy macrophages, sometimes accompanied by a T-cell-dominated inflammatory infiltrate (**Figure 13A**). These inflammatory processes drive active demyelination in adjacent parenchymal regions, where macrophages contain Luxol fast blue-positive myelin fragments and neutral lipids (**Figure 13B** and **C**).

Unlike MS, demyelination in ADEM primarily occurs around blood vessels, with axons largely preserved, though some may show signs of acute injury [140]. In more severe cases, fibrinous exudates may be present in vessel walls, and adjacent parenchymal necrosis can occur, demonstrating pathological similarities to AHLE.

A defining feature of classical ADEM is that perivenous demyelinating lesions tend to be of uniform histologic age, distinguishing it from MS, where lesions are typically distributed across different time points. These lesions can be widespread throughout the CNS or confined to a specific region, with a notable preference for white matter involvement. However, they may also involve the cortex, thalamus, and basal ganglia [125]. Commonly affected structures also include the spinal cord, brainstem, and cerebellum. ADEM is typically characterized by small, non-confluent perivenous lesions that differentiate it from the larger confluent perivenous plaques of MS [140].

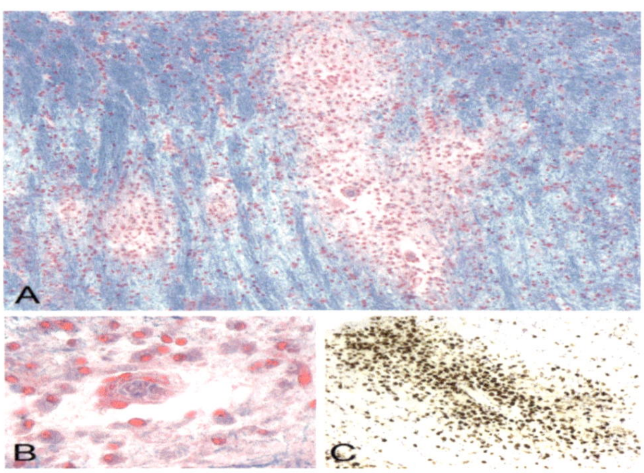

Figure 13.
Histopathological Features of Acute Disseminated Encephalomyelitis (ADEM) [139] (A) Luxol fast blue (LFB) staining shows characteristic small perivenous demyelinating lesions. (B) High-magnification LFB staining reveals macrophages containing LFB-positive degradation products. (C) CD68 immunostaining highlights numerous macrophages involved in the demyelination process. Magnifications: A, C (×100); B (×600).

1.8.3.3.4 Antibodies and ADEM

The presence of anti- MOG antibodies has been increasingly recognized in a subset of pediatric patients with ADEM [141]. These individuals tend to have a relapsing disease course. Additionally, they display an increased frequency of optic neuritis, longitudinally extensive transverse myelitis (LETM), or brainstem involvement, often manifesting with intractable hiccups or vomiting. The long-term neurological prognosis in anti-MOG-associated ADEM appears to be worse compared to MOG-negative cases, suggesting that antibody status may play a critical role in disease classification and prognosis.

1.8.4 Clinical variants of ADEM

Historically, the absence of uniform diagnostic criteria has led to the misclassification of various CNS demyelinating events under the umbrella of ADEM [135]. To address this, an international panel has proposed standardized definitions for acquired CNS DDs, distinguishing monophasic and relapsing variants of ADEM [111]:

1. *ADEM*: A first clinical, self-limiting demyelinating event characterized by acute or subacute encephalopathy with polyfocal deficits and widespread not pre-existing hyperintense lesions predominantly affecting CNS white matter.

2. *Recurrent disseminated encephalomyelitis (RDEM)*: Defined by an initial ADEM episode followed by another event fulfilling ADEM diagnostic criteria, occurring at least 3 months after the first episode and 4 weeks after completing steroid therapy, reproducing the original clinical syndrome.

3. *Multiphasic disseminated encephalomyelitis (MDEM)*: Characterized by one or more relapses of ADEM, each featuring encephalopathy and multifocal deficits but affecting new CNS regions on MRI and neurological examination, at least 3 months after the initial ADEM episode and 4 weeks after completing steroid therapy.

1.8.5 Differential diagnosis of ADEM

The coexistence of acute encephalopathy and CNS demyelination poses a considerable diagnostic challenge. Numerous inflammatory and non-inflammatory conditions can present with overlapping clinical and radiological features, necessitating thorough evaluation to ensure accurate differentiation and appropriate management.

The differential diagnosis for ADEM [142] includes:

- *Aseptic meningitis and acute viral encephalitis* often present with constitutional symptoms indicative of an underlying infection, including fever, neck rigidity, and elevated acute-phase reactants such as C-reactive protein and erythrocyte sedimentation rate.

- *The first clinical attack of MS*, where multifocal neurological deficits and MRI findings may resemble ADEM. However, MS relapses typically do not present with acute encephalopathy.

- *MOG antibody disease (MOGAD)*, which especially affects children and may mimic ADEM [107, 143].
- *Brain metastasis.*
- *Brucellosis.*
- *Cardioembolic stroke.*
- *Cauda equina and conus medullaris syndrome.*
- *Cavernous sinus syndromes.*
- *CNS complications in human immunodeficiency virus (HIV).*
- *Cerebral venous thrombosis.*
- *Churg-Strauss disease.*

Diagnosing ADEM is generally more straightforward when it follows an exanthem or immunization, as the presence of a latent period between systemic symptoms and neurological illness supports ADEM. The characteristic pattern of diffuse and multifocal involvement in both the central and peripheral nervous system, along with the typical MRI appearance, aids in distinguishing ADEM from other conditions.

One of the most critical questions in ADEM diagnosis is whether it can be definitively distinguished from the initial manifestation of MS [144–146]. A study by Schwarz et al. involving 40 patients initially diagnosed with ADEM found that 35% later developed clinically definite MS (as per Poser's criteria) over an average

• Multiple sclerosis
• Vasculitis
• Reversible posterior leucoencephalopathy
• Eclampsia
• Subcortical arteriosclerotic leucoencephalopathy
• Neurosarcoidosis
• Progressive multifocal leucoencephalopathy
• HIV encephalopathy
• Subacute sclerosing panencephalitis
• Mitochondrial encephalopathy
• Leucodystrophies
• Toxic encephalopathies
• Osmotic myelinolysis
• Aging

Table 3.
Causes of patchy areas of increased signal intensity in T2-weighted images on MRI [44].

follow-up of 38 months [147]. Hynson et al. highlighted that distinguishing ADEM from an initial MS attack in children can be difficult, but certain features—such as a preceding viral illness, early-onset ataxia, higher lesion load on MRI, involvement of deep cortical gray matter, and the absence of oligoclonal bands—favor an ADEM diagnosis [115].

Currently, distinguishing MS from ADEM based on a single MRI examination is not possible. Serial imaging performed at least 6 months apart is more useful. The appearance of new lesions on follow-up MRIs is highly suggestive of MS or clinical relapse in ADEM [148]. In monophasic demyelinating diseases like ADEM, MS should not be diagnosed unless new symptoms or imaging abnormalities appear more than 3 months after onset [144, 146, 149].

MRI features in DDs can overlap with antiphospholipid syndrome, making differentiation challenging. Cuadrado et al. suggested that a thorough medical history, previous thrombotic events, fetal loss history, abnormal MRI lesion localization, and response to anticoagulant therapy may assist in distinguishing these two conditions [150].

Epidemic CNS symptoms, absence of focal neurological signs, and persistent systemic involvement are more suggestive of viral encephalitis [144]. In endemic regions, ADEM should also be differentiated from *post-malarial neurological syndrome (PMNS)* [151, 152]. ADEM and PMNS share a lot of clinical and imaging similarities. Mohsen et al. proposed that ADEM and PMNS are indistinguishable, suggesting that *P. falciparum* should be considered a potential ADEM trigger.

On MRI, multiple patchy hyperintensities in the subcortical white matter on conventional T2-weighted, proton density-weighted, and FLAIR sequences have an extensive differential diagnosis (**Table 3**) [148].

1.8.6 Treatment of ADEM

Currently, there is no standardized therapy for ADEM, and treatment strategies have been derived from expert consensus. Supportive care during the acute phase is essential, with early initiation of antiviral therapy, such as acyclovir (30 mg/kg/day), strongly recommended at admission. This is because viral encephalitis, particularly herpes simplex encephalitis, is a common initial differential diagnosis in children.

The mainstay of ADEM treatment involves a short course (3–5 days) of intravenous corticosteroids, typically methylprednisolone (20–30 mg/kg/day, up to a maximum dose of 1 g/day) or dexamethasone (1 mg/kg/day), followed by a gradual taper of oral prednisone over 4–6 weeks [115, 116, 125, 135, 153].

IVIg has been utilized as either a second-line treatment in steroid-resistant cases or as an adjunct to corticosteroid therapy. The recommended IVIg regimen is 2 g/kg, administered over 2–5 days.

Plasmapheresis has emerged as a potential escalation therapy for severe or steroid-refractory ADEM. While its use is well-documented in acute fulminant CNS demyelinating diseases, its application in ADEM remains limited to small case reports.

AHLE, considered the most aggressive form of ADEM, has historically had a universally fatal course within hours to days if untreated. However, survival has been documented in pediatric patients treated with an aggressive multimodal approach, including high-dose corticosteroids, IVIg, plasmapheresis, and surgical decompression.

In cases of fulminant ADEM with uncontrolled intracranial pressure, when conventional medical management and critical care interventions fail to stabilize the patient, surgical decompression may be required.

1.8.7 Prognosis and outcome of ADEM

The prognosis of ADEM is highly variable and influenced by factors such as patient age, clinical severity, MRI findings, and the presence of MOG antibodies. Severe cases, particularly those classified as acute hemorrhagic encephalitis or acute necrotizing leukoencephalitis, have reported mortality rates as high as 30%. The prognosis is also affected by the underlying infection that triggered ADEM. Historically, cases following measles infection had significantly worse outcomes compared to those associated with other infections.

Approximately 25% of pediatric ADEM patients require intensive care admission, with an overall mortality rate of 1–3%. Adult patients experience a higher rate of ICU admission, longer hospital stays, poorer recovery, and greater mortality compared to children. While long-term neurological deficits are uncommon, cognitive impairment has been reported in up to 56% of children following ADEM [153, 154].

Full recovery from ADEM typically occurs within 1–6 months. Recovery rates vary, with 57–89% of patients regaining full neurological function after a single ADEM episode. However, 20–30% of individuals may develop minor residual deficits. The most commonly reported long-term impairments include: (a) Focal motor deficits, ranging from mild coordination difficulties to severe hemiparesis. (b) Visual disturbances, ranging from reduced visual acuity to complete blindness. (c) The development of seizures post-ADEM resolution [125].

2. Conclusions

Idiopathic inflammatory DDs of the CNS include several diseases, of which MS is the most common. Atypical inflammatory demyelinating syndromes are rare disorders that have pathological features similar to those seen in MS but differ from MS owing to unusual clinical or imaging manifestations or poor response to treatments used for MS. These syndromes include NMOSD, ADEM, TD, BCS, Schilder's disease, and Marburg's MS.

The substantial overlap in clinical presentation and imaging findings among these disorders presents a significant diagnostic challenge. Accurate identification is crucial, as management strategies vary considerably between MS and its atypical variants. Advances in neuroimaging, neuropathology, and immunological research are essential to further delineate these syndromes, establish clearer diagnostic criteria, and determine their potential interrelationships. A deeper understanding of these conditions will not only refine diagnostic precision but also facilitate the development of targeted therapies, ultimately improving patient outcomes.

Author details

Eleni Litsou
University Hospital of Ioannina, Greece

*Address all correspondence to: elenilitsou@gmail.com

References

[1] Hardy TA. Pseudotumoral demyelinating lesions: Diagnostic approach and long-term outcome. Current Opinion in Neurology. 2019;**32**(3):467-474. DOI: 10.1097/WCO.0000000000000683

[2] Comi G. Multiple sclerosis: Pseudotumoral forms. Neurological Sciences. 2004;**25**(Suppl. 4):S374-S379. DOI: 10.1007/s10072-004-0345-x

[3] van der Velden M, Bots GT, Endtz LJ. Cranial CT in multiple sclerosis showing a mass effect. Surgical Neurology. 1979;**12**(4):307-310

[4] Lucchinetti CF, Gavrilova RH, Metz I, et al. Clinical and radiographic spectrum of pathologically confirmed tumefactive multiple sclerosis. Brain. 2008;**131**(Pt 7):1759-1775. DOI: 10.1093/brain/awn098

[5] Kiriyama T, Kataoka H, Taoka T, et al. Characteristic neuroimaging in patients with tumefactive demyelinating lesions exceeding 30 mm. Journal of Neuroimaging. 2011;**21**(2):e69-e77. DOI: 10.1111/j.1552-6569.2010. 00502.x

[6] Enzinger C, Strasser-Fuchs S, Ropele S, Kapeller P, Kleinert R, Fazekas F. Tumefactive demyelinating lesions: Conventional and advanced magnetic resonance imaging. Multiple Sclerosis. 2005;**11**(2):135-139. DOI: 10.1191/1352458505ms1145oa

[7] Zagzag D, Miller DC, Kleinman GM, Abati A, Donnenfeld H, Budzilovich GN. Demyelinating disease versus tumor in surgical neuropathology. Clues to a correct pathological diagnosis. The American Journal of Surgical Pathology. 1993;**17**(6):537-545. DOI: 10.1097/00000478-199306000-00001

[8] Peterson K, Rosenblum MK, Powers JM, Alvord E, Walker RW, Posner JB. Effect of brain irradiation on demyelinating lesions. Neurology. 1993;**43**(10):2105-2112. DOI: 10.1212/wnl.43.10.2105

[9] Hunter SB, Ballinger WE Jr, Rubin JJ. Multiple sclerosis mimicking primary brain tumor. Archives of Pathology & Laboratory Medicine. 1987;**111**(5):464-468

[10] Kuan YC, Wang KC, Yuan WH, Tsai CP. Tumefactive multiple sclerosis in Taiwan. PLoS One. 2013;**8**(7):e69919. DOI: 10.1371/journal.pone.0069919

[11] Altintas A, Petek B, Isik N, et al. Clinical and radiological characteristics of tumefactive demyelinating lesions: Follow-up study. Multiple Sclerosis. 2012;**18**(10):1448-1453. DOI: 10.1177/1352458512438237

[12] Qi W, Jia GE, Wang X, Zhang M, Ma Z. Cerebral tumefactive demyelinating lesions. Oncology Letters. 2015;**10**(3):1763-1768. DOI: 10.3892/ol.2015.3481. Epub 2015 Jul 10

[13] Dagher AP, Smirniotopoulos J. Tumefactive demyelinating lesions. Neuroradiology. 1996;**38**(6):560-565. DOI: 10.1007/BF00626098

[14] Masdeu JC, Quinto C, Olivera C, Tenner M, Leslie D, Visintainer P. Open-ring imaging sign: Highly specific for atypical brain demyelination. Neurology. 2000;**54**(7):1427-1433. DOI: 10.1212/wnl.54.7.1427

[15] Klawiter EC, Benzinger T, Roy A, Naismith RT, Parks BJ, Cross AH. Spinal cord ring enhancement in multiple sclerosis. Archives of Neurology. 2010;**67**(11):1395-1398. DOI: 10.1001/archneurol.2010.271

[16] Given CA 2nd, Stevens BS, Lee C. The MRI appearance of tumefactive demyelinating lesions. AJR. American Journal of Roentgenology. 2004;**182**(1):195-199. DOI: 10.2214/ajr.182.1.1820195

[17] He J, Grossman RI, Ge Y, Mannon LJ. Enhancing patterns in multiple sclerosis: Evolution and persistence. AJNR. American Journal of Neuroradiology. 2001;**22**(4):664-669

[18] Crooks V, Waller S, Smith T, Hahn TJ. The use of the Karnofsky Performance Scale in determining outcomes and risk in geriatric outpatients. Journal of Gerontology. 1991;**46**(4):M139-M144. DOI: 10.1093/geronj/46.4.m139

[19] Mitha AP, Scott JN, George D, Hanson A, MacRae ME, Bell RB. Tumefactive demyelinating lesions. The Canadian Journal of Neurological Sciences. 2007;**34**(3):362-364. DOI: 10.1017/s0317167100006831

[20] Kim DS, Na DG, Kim KH, et al. Distinguishing tumefactive demyelinating lesions from glioma or central nervous system lymphoma: Added value of unenhanced CT compared with conventional contrast-enhanced MR imaging. Radiology. 2009;**251**(2):467-475. DOI: 10.1148/radiol.2512072071

[21] Kuhlmann T, Lassmann H, Brück W. Diagnosis of inflammatory demyelination in biopsy specimens: A practical approach. Acta Neuropathologica. 2008;**115**(3):275-287. DOI: 10.1007/s00401-007-0320-8

[22] Hardy TA, Reddel SW, Barnett MH, Palace J, Lucchinetti CF, Weinshenker BG. Atypical inflammatory demyelinating syndromes of the CNS. Lancet Neurology. 2016;**15**(9):967-981. DOI: 10.1016/S1474-4422(16)30043-6

[23] Cha S, Pierce S, Knopp EA, et al. Dynamic contrast-enhanced T2*-weighted MR imaging of tumefactive demyelinating lesions. AJNR. American Journal of Neuroradiology. 2001;**22**(6):1109-1116

[24] Weinshenker BG. Therapeutic plasma exchange for acute inflammatory demyelinating syndromes of the central nervous system. Journal of Clinical Apheresis. 1999;**14**(3):144-148. DOI: 10.1002/(sici)1098-1101(1999)14:3<144::aid-jca7>3.0.co;2-r

[25] Keegan M, Pineda AA, McClelland RL, Darby CH, Rodriguez M, Weinshenker BG. Plasma exchange for severe attacks of CNS demyelination: Predictors of response. Neurology. 2002;**58**(1):143-146. DOI: 10.1212/wnl.58.1.143

[26] CHAMPS Study Group. Interferon beta-1a for optic neuritis patients at high risk for multiple sclerosis. American Journal of Ophthalmology. 2001;**132**(4):463-471. DOI: 10.1016/s0002-9394(01)01209-0

[27] Confavreux C, Vukusic S. Natural history of multiple sclerosis: Implications for counselling and therapy. Current Opinion in Neurology. 2002;**15**(3):257-266. DOI: 10.1097/00019052-200206000-00006

[28] Karaarslan E, Altintas A, Senol U, Yeni N, Dincer A, Bayindir C, et al. Baló's concentric sclerosis: Clinical and

radiologic features of five cases. AJNR. American Journal of Neuroradiology. 2001;**22**(7):1362-1367. Available from: https://pmc.ncbi.nlm.nih.gov/articles/PMC7975204/

[29] Li Y, Xie P, Fan X, Tang H. Balò's concentric sclerosis presenting with benign clinical course and multiple sclerosis-like lesions on magnetic resonance images. Neurology India. 2009;**57**(1):66-68. DOI: 10.4103/0028-3886.48815

[30] Tabira T. Concentric sclerosis (Baló). Nihon Rinsho. 1994;**52**(11):2971-2975. Japanese. Available from: https://pubmed.ncbi.nlm.nih.gov/7996696/

[31] Mowry EM, Woo JH, Ances BM. Baló's concentric sclerosis presenting as a stroke-like syndrome. Nature Clinical Practice. Neurology. 2007;**3**(6):349-354. DOI: 10.1038/ncpneuro0522

[32] Hardy TA, Miller DH. Baló's concentric sclerosis. Lancet Neurology. 2014;**13**(7):740-746. DOI: 10.1016/S1474-4422(14)70052-3

[33] Jarius S, Würthwein C, Behrens JR, Wanner J, Haas J, Paul F, et al. Baló's concentric sclerosis is immunologically distinct from multiple sclerosis: Results from retrospective analysis of almost 150 lumbar punctures. Journal of Neuroinflammation. 2018;**15**(1):22. DOI: 10.1186/s12974-017-1043-y

[34] Marburg O. Acute multiple sclerosis (encephalomyelitis pariaxialis scleroticans). Journal of Psychiatry and Neurology. 1906;**27**:211-312

[35] Stadelmann C, Ludwin S, Tabira T, Guseo A, Lucchinetti CF, Leel-Ossy L, et al. Tissue preconditioning may explain concentric lesions in Baló's type of multiple sclerosis. Brain. 2005;**128**(Pt 5):979-987. DOI: 10.1093/brain/awh457. Epub 2005 Mar 17

[36] Kastrup O, Stude P, Limmroth V. Balo's concentric sclerosis. Evolution of active demyelination demonstrated by serial contrast-enhanced MRI. Journal of Neurology. 2002;**249**(7):811-814. DOI: 10.1007/s00415-002-0718-0

[37] Darke M, Bahador FM, Miller DC, Litofsky NS, Ahsan H. Baló's concentric sclerosis: Imaging findings and pathological correlation. Journal of Radiology Case Reports. 2013;**7**(6):1-8. DOI: 10.3941/jrcr. v7i6.1251

[38] Caracciolo JT, Murtagh RD, Rojiani AM, Murtagh FR. Pathognomonic MR imaging findings in Balo concentric sclerosis. AJNR. American Journal of Neuroradiology. 2001;**22**(2):292-293. Available from: https://pmc.ncbi.nlm.nih.gov/articles/PMC7973934/

[39] Wengert O, Siebert E. Images in clinical medicine. Baló's concentric sclerosis. The New England Journal of Medicine. 2011;**365**(8):742. DOI: 10.1056/NEJMicm1008401

[40] Kavanagh EC, Heran MK, Fenton DM, Lapointe JS, Nugent RA, Graeb DA. Diffusion-weighted imaging findings in Balo concentric sclerosis. The British Journal of Radiology. 2006;**79**(943):e28-e31. DOI: 10.1259/bjr/36636301

[41] Mowry EM, Woo JH, Ances BM. Technology insight: Can neuroimaging provide insights into the role of ischemia in Baló's concentric sclerosis? Nature Clinical Practice. Neurology. 2007;**3**(6):341-348. DOI: 10.1038/ncpneuro0519

[42] Kim MO, Lee SA, Choi CG, Huh JR, Lee MC. Balo's concentric

sclerosis: A clinical case study of brain MRI, biopsy, and proton magnetic resonance spectroscopic findings. Journal of Neurology, Neurosurgery, and Psychiatry. 1997;**62**(6):655-658. DOI: 10.1136/jnnp.62.6.655

[43] Popescu BF, Lucchinetti CF. Pathology of demyelinating diseases. Annual Review of Pathology. 2012;7:185-217. DOI: 10.1146/annurev-pathol-011811-132443

[44] Garg RK. Acute disseminated encephalomyelitis. Postgraduate Medical Journal. 2003;**79**(927):11-17. DOI: 10.1136/pmj.79.927.11

[45] Yao DL, Webster HD, Hudson LD, Brenner M, Liu DS, Escobar AI, et al. Concentric sclerosis (Baló): Morphometric and in situ hybridization study of lesions in six patients. Annals of Neurology. 1994;**35**(1):18-30. DOI: 10.1002/ana.410350105

[46] Lucchinetti C, Brück W, Parisi J, Scheithauer B, Rodriguez M, Lassmann H. Heterogeneity of multiple sclerosis lesions: Implications for the pathogenesis of demyelination. Annals of Neurology. 2000;**47**(6):707-717. DOI: 10.1002/1531-8249(200006)47:6<707::aid-ana3>3.0.co;2-q

[47] Schilder P. Zur ke nutnis der Sogenammten diffusen Sklerose (Über Encephalitis Periaxialis Diffusa). Z Ges Neurol Psychiatry. 1912;**10**:1-60. Available from: https://ia600607.us.archive.org/view_archive.php?archive=/8/items/crossref-pre-1923-scholarly-works/10.1007%252Fbf02895227.zip&file=10.1007%252Fbf02901445.pdf

[48] Lassmann H. Neuropathology in multiple sclerosis: New concepts. Multiple Sclerosis. 1998;**4**(3):93-98. DOI: 10.1177/135245859800400301

[49] Afifi AK, Follett KA, Greenlee J, Scott WE, Moore SA. Optic neuritis: A novel presentation of Schilder's disease. Journal of Child Neurology. 2001;**16**(9):693-696. DOI: 10.1177/088307380101600915

[50] Cañellas AR, Gols AR, Izquierdo JR, Subirana MT, Gairin XM. Idiopathic inflammatory-demyelinating diseases of the central nervous system. Neuroradiology. 2007;**49**(5):393-409. DOI: 10.1007/s00234-007-0216-2. Epub 2007 Feb 28

[51] Poser CM, Goutières F, Carpentier MA, Aicardi J. Schilder's myelinoclastic diffuse sclerosis. Pediatrics. 1986;**77**(1):107-112. Erratum in: Pediatrics 1986;78(1):138. Available from: https://pubmed.ncbi.nlm.nih.gov/3940347/

[52] Poser CM, Brinar VV. The nature of multiple sclerosis. Clinical Neurology and Neurosurgery. 2004;**106**(3):159-171. DOI: 10.1016/j.clineuro.2004.02.005

[53] Kim BJ, Kim B-J, Lee KH, Kim G-M. A Pathology-proven Case of Schilder's Disease. Journal of the Korean Neurological Association. 2008;**26**:50-54. Available from: https://api.semanticscholar.org/CorpusID:75392926

[54] Bacigaluppi S, Polonara G, Zavanone ML, Campanella R, Branca V, Gaini SM, et al. Schilder's disease: Non-invasive diagnosis?: A case report and review. Neurological Sciences. 2009;**30**(5):421-430. DOI: 10.1007/s10072-009-0113-z. Epub 2009 Jul 17

[55] Kurul S, Cakmakçi H, Dirik E, Kovanlikaya A. Schilder's disease: Case study with serial neuroimaging. Journal

of Child Neurology. 2003;**18**(1):58-61. DOI: 10.1177/08830738030180011301

[56] Fitzgerald MJ, Coleman LT. Recurrent myelinoclastic diffuse sclerosis: A case report of a child with Schilder's variant of multiple sclerosis. Pediatric Radiology. 2000 Dec;**30**(12):861-865. DOI: 10.1007/s002470000346

[57] Poppe M, Brück W, Hahn G, Weissbrich B, Heubner G, Goebel HH, et al. Fulminant course in a case of diffuse myelinoclastic encephalitis—A case report. Neuropediatrics. 2001;**32**(1):41-44. DOI: 10.1055/s-2001-12214

[58] Garrido C, Levy-Gomes A, Teixeira J, Temudo T. Enfermedad de Schilder: Dos nuevos casos y revisión de la bibliografía [Schilder's disease: Two new cases and a review of the literature]. Revista de Neurologia. 2004;**39**(8):734-738. Spanish. Available from: https://pubmed.ncbi.nlm.nih.gov/15514902/

[59] Garell PC, Menezes AH, Baumbach G, Moore SA, Nelson G, Mathews K, et al. Presentation, management and follow-up of Schilder's disease. Pediatric Neurosurgery. 1998;**29**(2):86-91. DOI: 10.1159/000028695

[60] Jarius S, Wildemann B. The history of neuromyelitis optica. Journal of Neuroinflammation. 2013;**10**:8. DOI: 10.1186/1742-2094-10-8

[61] Wingerchuk DM, Hogancamp WF, O'Brien PC, Weinshenker BG. The clinical course of neuromyelitis optica (Devic's syndrome). Neurology. 1999;**53**(5):1107-1114. DOI: 10.1212/wnl.53.5.1107

[62] Wingerchuk DM, Lennon VA, Lucchinetti CF, Pittock SJ, Weinshenker BG. The spectrum of neuromyelitis optica. Lancet Neurology. 2007;**6**(9):805-815. DOI: 10.1016/S1474-4422(07)70216-8

[63] Lennon VA, Wingerchuk DM, Kryzer TJ, Pittock SJ, Lucchinetti CF, Fujihara K, et al. A serum autoantibody marker of neuromyelitis optica: Distinction from multiple sclerosis. Lancet. 2004;**364**(9451):2106-2112. DOI: 10.1016/S0140-6736(04)17551-X

[64] Lennon VA, Kryzer TJ, Pittock SJ, Verkman AS, Hinson SR. IgG marker of optic-spinal multiple sclerosis binds to the aquaporin-4 water channel. The Journal of Experimental Medicine. 2005;**202**(4):473-477. DOI: 10.1084/jem.20050304. Epub 2005 Aug 8

[65] Wingerchuk DM, Lennon VA, Pittock SJ, Lucchinetti CF, Weinshenker BG. Revised diagnostic criteria for neuromyelitis optica. Neurology. 2006;**66**(10):1485-1489. DOI: 10.1212/01.wnl.0000216139.44259.74

[66] Wingerchuk DM. Neuromyelitis optica spectrum disorders. Continuum (Minneap Minn). 2010;**16**(5 Multiple Sclerosis):105-121. DOI: 10.1212/01.CON.0000389937.69413.15

[67] Wingerchuk DM, Banwell B, Bennett JL, Cabre P, Carroll W, Chitnis T, et al. International consensus diagnostic criteria for neuromyelitis optica spectrum disorders. Neurology. 2015;**85**(2):177-189. DOI: 10.1212/WNL.0000000000001729. Epub 2015 Jun 19

[68] Papadopoulos MC, Verkman AS. Aquaporin 4 and neuromyelitis optica. Lancet Neurology. 2012;**11**(6):535-544. DOI: 10.1016/S1474-4422(12)70133-3. Epub 2012 May 16

[69] Matiello M, Kim HJ, Kim W, Brum DG, Barreira AA, Kingsbury DJ, et al. Familial neuromyelitis optica. Neurology. 2010;**75**(4):310-315. DOI: 10.1212/WNL.0b013e3181ea9f15

[70] Tzartos JS, Stergiou C, Kilidireas K, Zisimopoulou P, Thomaidis T, Tzartos SJ. Anti-aquaporin-1 autoantibodies in patients with neuromyelitis optica spectrum disorders. PLoS One. 2013;**8**(9):e74773. DOI: 10.1371/journal.pone.0074773

[71] Jasiak-Zatonska M, Kalinowska-Lyszczarz A, Michalak S, Kozubski W. The immunology of neuromyelitis optica-current knowledge, clinical implications, controversies and future perspectives. International Journal of Molecular Sciences. 2016;**17**(3):273. DOI: 10.3390/ijms17030273

[72] Saadoun S, Waters P, Owens GP, Bennett JL, Vincent A, Papadopoulos MC. Neuromyelitis optica MOG-IgG causes reversible lesions in mouse brain. Acta Neuropathologica Communications. 2014;**2**:35. DOI: 10.1186/2051-5960-2-35

[73] McKeon A, Pittock SJ. Neuromyelitis optica and the evolving spectrum of water channel autoimmunity: A new direction. European Journal of Neurology. 2009;**16**(4):433-435. DOI: 10.1111/j.1468-1331.2008. 02385.x

[74] Lucchinetti CF, Mandler RN, McGavern D, Bruck W, Gleich G, Ransohoff RM, et al. A role for humoral mechanisms in the pathogenesis of Devic's neuromyelitis optica. Brain. 2002;**125**(Pt 7):1450-1461. DOI: 10.1093/brain/awf151

[75] Nakashima I, Fujihara K, Fujimori J, Narikawa K, Misu T, Itoyama Y. Absence of IgG1 response in the cerebrospinal fluid of relapsing neuromyelitis optica. Neurology. 2004;**62**(1):144-146. DOI: 10.1212/wnl.62.1.144

[76] Chang VTW, Chang HM. Review: Recent advances in the understanding of the pathophysiology of neuromyelitis optica spectrum disorder. Neuropathology and Applied Neurobiology. 2020;**46**(3):199-218. DOI: 10.1111/nan.12574. Epub 2019 Aug 14

[77] Mandler RN. Neuromyelitis optica - Devic's syndrome, update. Autoimmunity Reviews. 2006;**5**(8):537-543. DOI: 10.1016/j.autrev.2006.02.008. Epub 2006 Mar 21

[78] Pohl D, Waubant E, Banwell B, Chabas D, Chitnis T, Weinstock-Guttman B, et al. Treatment of pediatric multiple sclerosis and variants. Neurology. 2007;**68**(16 Suppl 2):S54-S65. DOI: 10.1212/01.wnl.0000259407.40023.ab

[79] Watanabe S, Nakashima I, Misu T, Miyazawa I, Shiga Y, Fujihara K, et al. Therapeutic efficacy of plasma exchange in NMO-IgG-positive patients with neuromyelitis optica. Multiple Sclerosis. 2007;**13**(1):128-132. DOI: 10.1177/1352458506071174

[80] O'Riordan JI, Gallagher HL, Thompson AJ, Howard RS, Kingsley DP, Thompson EJ, et al. Clinical, CSF, and MRI findings in Devic's neuromyelitis optica. Journal of Neurology, Neurosurgery, and Psychiatry. 1996;**60**(4):382-387. DOI: 10.1136/jnnp.60.4.382

[81] Cree BA, Lamb S, Morgan K, Chen A, Waubant E, Genain C. An open label study of the effects of rituximab in neuromyelitis optica. Neurology. 2005;**64**(7):1270-1272. DOI: 10.1212/01.WNL.0000159399.81861.D5

[82] Warabi Y, Matsumoto Y, Hayashi H. Interferon beta-1b exacerbates multiple sclerosis with severe optic nerve and spinal cord demyelination. Journal of the Neurological Sciences. 2007;**252**(1):57-61. DOI: 10.1016/j.jns.2006.10.008. Epub 2006 Nov 27

[83] Tradtrantip L, Zhang H, Saadoun S, Phuan PW, Lam C, Papadopoulos MC, et al. Anti-aquaporin-4 monoclonal antibody blocker therapy for neuromyelitis optica. Annals of Neurology. 2012;**71**(3):314-322. DOI: 10.1002/ana.22657. Epub 2012 Jan 23

[84] Saadoun S, Waters P, MacDonald C, Bell BA, Vincent A, Verkman AS, et al. Neutrophil protease inhibition reduces neuromyelitis optica-immunoglobulin G-induced damage in mouse brain. Annals of Neurology. 2012;**71**(3):323-333. DOI: 10.1002/ana.22686. Epub 2012 Feb 28

[85] Pittock SJ, Lennon VA, McKeon A, Mandrekar J, Weinshenker BG, Lucchinetti CF, et al. Eculizumab in AQP4-IgG-positive relapsing neuromyelitis optica spectrum disorders: An open-label pilot study. Lancet Neurology. 2013;**12**(6):554-562. DOI: 10.1016/S1474-4422(13)70076-0. Epub 2013 Apr 26

[86] Araki M, Matsuoka T, Miyamoto K, Kusunoki S, Okamoto T, Murata M, et al. Efficacy of the anti-IL-6 receptor antibody tocilizumab in neuromyelitis optica: A pilot study. Neurology. 2014;**82**(15):1302-1306. DOI: 10.1212/WNL.0000000000000317. Epub 2014 Mar 14

[87] Johnson MD, Lavin P, Whetsell WO Jr. Fulminant monophasic multiple sclerosis, Marburg's type. Journal of Neurology, Neurosurgery, and Psychiatry. 1990;**53**(10):918-921. DOI: 10.1136/jnnp.53.10.918

[88] Jeffery DR, Lefkowitz DS, Crittenden JP. Treatment of Marburg variant multiple sclerosis with mitoxantrone. Journal of Neuroimaging. 2004;**14**(1):58-62

[89] Walid MS, Sanoufa M. The diagnosis of Marburg disease is course-dependent. GMS German Medical Science. 2010;**8**:Doc06. DOI: 10.3205/000095

[90] Hu W, Lucchinetti CF. The pathological spectrum of CNS inflammatory demyelinating diseases. Seminars in Immunopathology. 2009;**31**(4):439-453. DOI: 10.1007/s00281-009-0178-z. Epub 2009 Sep 25

[91] Prineas JW, Kwon EE, Goldenberg PZ, Ilyas AA, Quarles RH, Benjamins JA, et al. Multiple sclerosis. Oligodendrocyte proliferation and differentiation in fresh lesions. Laboratory Investigation. 1989;**61**(5):489-503. Available from: https://pubmed.ncbi.nlm.nih.gov/2811298/

[92] Capello E, Mancardi GL. Marburg type and Balò's concentric sclerosis: Rare and acute variants of multiple sclerosis. Neurological Sciences. 2004;**25**(Suppl 4):S361-S363. DOI: 10.1007/s10072-004-0341-1

[93] Harauz G, Ishiyama N, Hill CM, Bates IR, Libich DS, Farès C. Myelin basic protein-diverse conformational states of an intrinsically unstructured protein and its roles in myelin assembly and multiple sclerosis. Micron. 2004;**35**(7):503-542. DOI: 10.1016/j.micron.2004.04.005

[94] Wood DD, Bilbao JM, O'Connors P, Moscarello MA. Acute multiple sclerosis (Marburg type) is associated with developmentally immature myelin basic protein. Annals of Neurology. 1996 Jul;**40**(1):18-24. DOI: 10.1002/ana.410400106

[95] Beniac DR, Wood DD, Palaniyar N, Ottensmeyer FP, Moscarello MA, Harauz G. Marburg's variant of multiple sclerosis correlates with a less compact structure of myelin basic protein. Molecular Cell Biology Research Communications. 1999 Apr;**1**(1):48-51. DOI: 10.1006/mcbr.1999.0111

[96] Manuel A, Vasudevan MC. A case of Marburg's variant of multiple sclerosis successfully treated with IVIg and mitoxantrone. Annals of Indian Academy of Neurology. 2021;**24**(1):92-94. DOI: 10.4103/aian.AIAN_117_20. Epub 2021 Feb 16

[97] Stadelmann C, Brück W. Lessons from the neuropathology of atypical forms of multiple sclerosis. Neurological Sciences. 2004;**25**(Suppl 4):S319-S322. DOI: 10.1007/s10072-004-0333-1

[98] Aliaga ES, Barkhof F. MRI mimics of multiple sclerosis. Handbook of Clinical Neurology. 2014;**122**:291-316. DOI: 10.1016/B978-0-444-52001-2.00012-1

[99] de Seze J, Debouverie M, Zephir H, Lebrun C, Blanc F, Bourg V, et al. Acute fulminant demyelinating disease: A descriptive study of 60 patients. Archives of Neurology. 2007;**64**(10):1426-1432. DOI: 10.1001/archneur.64.10.1426

[100] Kesselring J, Miller DH, Robb SA, Kendall BE, Moseley IF, Kingsley D, et al. Acute disseminated encephalomyelitis. MRI findings and the distinction from multiple sclerosis. Brain. 1990;**113**(Pt 2):291-302. DOI: 10.1093/brain/113.2.291

[101] Habek M, Barun B, Puretić Z, Brinar VV. Treatment of steroid unresponsive relapse with plasma exchange in aggressive multiple sclerosis. Therapeutic Apheresis and Dialysis. 2010;**14**(3):298-302. DOI: 10.1111/j.1744-9987.2009. 00794.x

[102] Neuhaus O, Kieseier BC, Hartung HP. Therapeutic role of mitoxantrone in multiple sclerosis. Pharmacology & Therapeutics. 2006;**109**(1-2):198-209. DOI: 10.1016/j.pharmthera.2005.07.002. Epub 2005 Aug 10

[103] Nozaki K, Abou-Fayssal N. High dose cyclophosphamide treatment in Marburg variant multiple sclerosis A case report. Journal of the Neurological Sciences. 2010;**296**(1-2):121-123. DOI: 10.1016/j.jns.2010.05.022. Epub 2010 Jun 25

[104] Menge T, Hemmer B, Nessler S, Wiendl H, Neuhaus O, Hartung HP, et al. Acute disseminated encephalomyelitis: An update. Archives of Neurology. 2005;**62**(11):1673-1680. DOI: 10.1001/archneur.62.11.1673

[105] Marchioni E, Ravaglia S, Piccolo G, Furione M, Zardini E, Franciotta D, et al. Postinfectious inflammatory disorders: Subgroups based on prospective follow-up. Neurology. 2005;**65**(7):1057-1065. DOI: 10.1212/01.wnl.0000179302.93960.ad

[106] Koelman DL, Mateen FJ. Acute disseminated encephalomyelitis: Current controversies in diagnosis and outcome. Journal of Neurology. 2015;**262**(9):2013-2024. DOI: 10.1007/s00415-015-7694-7. Epub 2015 Mar 13

[107] Paolilo RB, Deiva K, Neuteboom R, Rostásy K, Lim M. Acute disseminated encephalomyelitis: Current perspectives. Children (Basel). 2020;**7**(11):210. DOI: 10.3390/children7110210

[108] Leake JA, Albani S, Kao AS, Senac MO, Billman GF, Nespeca MP, et al. Acute disseminated encephalomyelitis in childhood: Epidemiologic,

clinical and laboratory features. The Pediatric Infectious Disease Journal. 2004;**23**(8):756-764. DOI: 10.1097/01.inf.0000133048.75452.dd

[109] Alper G, Heyman R, Wang L. Multiple sclerosis and acute disseminated encephalomyelitis diagnosed in children after long-term follow-up: Comparison of presenting features. Developmental Medicine and Child Neurology. 2009;**51**(6):480-486. DOI: 10.1111/j.1469-8749.2008. 03136.x. Epub 2008 Oct 24

[110] Wender M. Acute disseminated encephalomyelitis (ADEM). Journal of Neuroimmunology. 2011;**231**(1-2):92-99. DOI: 10.1016/j.jneuroim.2010.09.019. Epub 2011 Jan 14

[111] Krupp LB, Tardieu M, Amato MP, Banwell B, Chitnis T, Dale RC, et al. International Pediatric Multiple Sclerosis Study Group criteria for pediatric multiple sclerosis and immune-mediated central nervous system demyelinating disorders: Revisions to the 2007 definitions. Multiple Sclerosis. 2013;**19**(10):1261-1267. DOI: 10.1177/1352458513484547. Epub 2013 Apr 9

[112] Alves JM, Marques IB, Gil-Gouveia R. Controvérsias da Vacinação: A Propósito de Um Caso de Encefalomielite Aguda Disseminada em Adulto [Vaccination Controversies: An Adult Case of Post-Vaccinal Acute Disseminated Encephalomyelitis]. Acta Medica Portuguesa. 2019;**32**(1):81-85. DOI: 10.20344/amp.9809. Portuguese. Epub 2019 Feb 1

[113] Rossor T, Benetou C, Wright S, Duignan S, Lascelles K, Robinson R, et al. Early predictors of epilepsy and subsequent relapse in children with acute disseminated encephalomyelitis. Multiple Sclerosis. 2020;**26**(3):333-342. DOI: 10.1177/1352458518823486. Epub 2019 Feb 7

[114] Galetta KM, Bhattacharyya S. Multiple sclerosis and autoimmune neurology of the central nervous system. The Medical Clinics of North America. 2019;**103**(2):325-336. DOI: 10.1016/j.mcna.2018.10.004. Epub 2018 Dec 3

[115] Hynson JL, Kornberg AJ, Coleman LT, Shield L, Harvey AS, Kean MJ. Clinical and neuroradiologic features of acute disseminated encephalomyelitis in children. Neurology. 2001;**56**(10):1308-1312. DOI: 10.1212/wnl.56.10.1308

[116] Dale RC, de Sousa C, Chong WK, Cox TC, Harding B, Neville BG. Acute disseminated encephalomyelitis, multiphasic disseminated encephalomyelitis and multiple sclerosis in children. Brain. 2000;**123**(Pt 12):2407-2422. DOI: 10.1093/brain/123.12.2407

[117] Karussis D, Petrou P. The spectrum of post-vaccination inflammatory CNS demyelinating syndromes. Autoimmunity Reviews. 2014;**13**(3):215-224. DOI: 10.1016/j.autrev.2013.10.003

[118] Tenembaum SN. Acute disseminated encephalomyelitis. Handbook of Clinical Neurology. 2013;**112**:1253-1262. DOI: 10.1016/B978-0-444-52910-7.00048-9

[119] Dale RC, Church AJ, Cardoso F, Goddard E, Cox TC, Chong WK, et al. Poststreptococcal acute disseminated encephalomyelitis with basal ganglia involvement and auto-reactive antibasal ganglia antibodies. Annals of Neurology. 2001;**50**(5):588-595. DOI: 10.1002/ana.1250

[120] O'Connor KC, McLaughlin KA, De Jager PL, Chitnis T, Bettelli E, Xu C, et al. Self-antigen tetramers discriminate between myelin autoantibodies to native or

denatured protein. Nature Medicine. 2007;**13**(2):211-217. DOI: 10.1038/nm1488. Epub 2007 Jan 12

[121] Dale RC, Brilot F. Biomarkers of inflammatory and auto-immune central nervous system disorders. Current Opinion in Pediatrics. 2010;**22**(6):718-725. DOI: 10.1097/MOP.0b013e3283402b71

[122] Pröbstel AK, Dornmair K, Bittner R, Sperl P, Jenne D, Magalhaes S, et al. Antibodies to MOG are transient in childhood acute disseminated encephalomyelitis. Neurology. 2011;**77**(6):580-588. DOI: 10.1212/WNL.0b013e318228c0b1. Epub 2011 Jul 27

[123] Menge T, Kieseier BC, Nessler S, Hemmer B, Hartung HP, Stüve O. Acute disseminated encephalomyelitis: An acute hit against the brain. Current Opinion in Neurology. 2007;**20**(3):247-254. DOI: 10.1097/WCO.0b013e3280f31b45

[124] Wingerchuk DM, Lucchinetti CF. Comparative immunopathogenesis of acute disseminated encephalomyelitis, neuromyelitis optica, and multiple sclerosis. Current Opinion in Neurology. 2007;**20**(3):343-350. DOI: 10.1097/WCO.0b013e3280be58d8

[125] Tenembaum S, Chamoles N, Fejerman N. Acute disseminated encephalomyelitis: A long-term follow-up study of 84 pediatric patients. Neurology. 2002;**59**(8):1224-1231. DOI: 10.1212/wnl.59.8.1224

[126] Pohl D, Alper G, Van Haren K, Kornberg AJ, Lucchinetti CF, Tenembaum S, et al. Acute disseminated encephalomyelitis: Updates on an inflammatory CNS syndrome. Neurology. 2016;**87**(9 Suppl 2):S38-S45. DOI: 10.1212/WNL.0000000000002825

[127] Ketelslegers IA, Visser IE, Neuteboom RF, Boon M, Catsman-Berrevoets CE, Hintzen RQ. Disease course and outcome of acute disseminated encephalomyelitis is more severe in adults than in children. Multiple Sclerosis. 2011;**17**(4):441-448. DOI: 10.1177/1352458510390068. Epub 2010 Dec 8

[128] Li K, Li M, Wen L, Wang Q, Ding X, Wang J. Clinical presentation and outcomes of acute disseminated encephalomyelitis in adults worldwide: Systematic review and meta-analysis. Frontiers in Immunology. 2022;**13**:870867. DOI: 10.3389/fimmu.2022.870867

[129] Lee YJ. Acute disseminated encephalomyelitis in children: Differential diagnosis from multiple sclerosis on the basis of clinical course. Korean Journal of Pediatrics. 2011;**54**(6):234-240. DOI: 10.3345/kjp.2011.54.6.234. Epub 2011 Jun 30

[130] Lu Z, Zhang B, Qiu W, Kang Z, Shen L, Long Y, et al. Comparative brain stem lesions on MRI of acute disseminated encephalomyelitis, neuromyelitis optica, and multiple sclerosis. PLoS One. 2011;**6**(8):e22766. DOI: 10.1371/journal.pone.0022766. Epub 2011 Aug 10

[131] Kawanaka Y, Ando K, Ishikura R, Katsuura T, Wakata Y, Kodama H, et al. Delayed appearance of transient hyperintensity foci on T1-weighted magnetic resonance imaging in acute disseminated encephalomyelitis. Japanese Journal of Radiology. 2019;**37**(4):277-282. DOI: 10.1007/s11604-018-00808-w. Epub 2019 Jan 22

[132] Anand KS, Agrawal AK, Garg J, Dhamija RK, Mahajan RK. Spectrum of neurological complications in chikungunya fever: Experience at

a tertiary care centre and review of literature. Tropical Doctor. 2019;**49**(2):79-84. DOI: 10.1177/0049475518825219. Epub 2019 Jan 24

[133] Codjia P, Ayrignac X, Carra-Dalliere C, Cohen M, Charif M, Lippi A, et al. Multiple sclerosis with atypical MRI presentation: Results of a nationwide multicenter study in 57 consecutive cases. Multiple Sclerosis and Related Disorders. 2019;**28**:109-116. DOI: 10.1016/j.msard.2018.12.022. Epub 2018 Dec 18

[134] Ketelslegers IA, Neuteboom RF, Boon M, Catsman-Berrevoets CE, Hintzen RQ, Dutch Pediatric MS Study Group. A comparison of MRI criteria for diagnosing pediatric ADEM and MS. Neurology. 2010;**74**(18):1412-1415. DOI: 10.1212/WNL.0b013e3181dc138b. Epub 2010 Mar 24

[135] Tenembaum S, Chitnis T, Ness J, Hahn JS, International Pediatric MS Study Group. Acute disseminated encephalomyelitis. Neurology. 2007;**68**(16 Suppl 2):S23-S36. DOI: 10.1212/01.wnl.0000259404.51352.7f

[136] McDonald WI, Compston A, Edan G, Goodkin D, Hartung HP, Lublin FD, et al. Recommended diagnostic criteria for multiple sclerosis: Guidelines from the International Panel on the diagnosis of multiple sclerosis. Annals of Neurology. 2001;**50**(1):121-127. DOI: 10.1002/ana.1032

[137] Murthy JM, Yangala R, Meena AK, Jaganmohan RJ. Acute disseminated encephalomyelitis: Clinical and MRI study from South India. Journal of the Neurological Sciences. 1999;**165**(2):133-138. DOI: 10.1016/s0022-510x(99)00094-5

[138] Höllinger P, Sturzenegger M, Mathis J, Schroth G, Hess CW. Acute disseminated encephalomyelitis in adults: A reappraisal of clinical, CSF, EEG, and MRI findings. Journal of Neurology. 2002;**249**(3):320-329. DOI: 10.1007/s004150200012

[139] Höftberger R, Lassmann H. Inflammatory demyelinating diseases of the central nervous system. Handbook of Clinical Neurology. 2017;**145**:263-283. DOI: 10.1016/B978-0-12-802395-2.00019-5

[140] Young NP, Weinshenker BG, Parisi JE, Scheithauer B, Giannini C, Roemer SF, et al. Perivenous demyelination: Association with clinically defined acute disseminated encephalomyelitis and comparison with pathologically confirmed multiple sclerosis. Brain. 2010;**133**(Pt 2):333-348. DOI: 10.1093/brain/awp321. Epub 2010 Feb 3

[141] Armangue T, Olivé-Cirera G, Martínez-Hernandez E, Sepulveda M, Ruiz-Garcia R, Muñoz-Batista M, et al. Associations of paediatric demyelinating and encephalitic syndromes with myelin oligodendrocyte glycoprotein antibodies: A multicentre observational study. Lancet Neurology. 2020;**19**(3):234-246. Epub 2020 Feb 10. Erratum in: Lancet Neurol. 2020;19(4): e4. DOI: 10.1016/S1474-4422(19)30488-0

[142] Anilkumar AC, Foris LA, Tadi P. Acute disseminated encephalomyelitis. 2024. In: StatPearls [Internet]. Treasure Island (FL): StatPearls Publishing. p. 2025

[143] Ketelslegers IA, Van Pelt DE, Bryde S, Neuteboom RF, Catsman-Berrevoets CE, Hamann D, et al. Anti-MOG antibodies plead against MS diagnosis in an Acquired Demyelinating Syndromes cohort. Multiple Sclerosis. 2015;**21**(12):1513-1520. DOI: 10.1177/1352458514566666. Epub 2015 Feb 6

[144] Hartung HP, Grossman RI. ADEM: Distinct disease or part of the MS spectrum? Neurology. 2001;**56**(10):1257-1260. DOI: 10.1212/wnl.56.10.1257. Erratum in: Neurology 2001;57(6):1146

[145] Singh S, Prabhakar S, Korah IP, Warade SS, Alexander M. Acute disseminated encephalomyelitis and multiple sclerosis: Magnetic resonance imaging differentiation. Australasian Radiology. 2000;**44**(4):404-411. DOI: 10.1046/j.1440-1673.2000.00845.x

[146] Barkhof F, Filippi M, Miller DH, Scheltens P, Campi A, Polman CH, et al. Comparison of MRI criteria at first presentation to predict conversion to clinically definite multiple sclerosis. Brain. 1997;**120**(Pt 11):2059-2069. DOI: 10.1093/brain/120.11.2059

[147] Schwarz S, Mohr A, Knauth M, Wildemann B, Storch-Hagenlocher B. Acute disseminated encephalomyelitis: A follow-up study of 40 adult patients. Neurology. 2001;**56**(10):1313-1318. DOI: 10.1212/wnl.56.10.1313

[148] Stüve O, Zamvil SS. Pathogenesis, diagnosis, and treatment of acute disseminated encephalomyelitis. Current Opinion in Neurology. 1999;**12**(4):395-401. DOI: 10.1097/00019052-199908000-00005

[149] Hung KL, Liao HT, Tsai ML. Postinfectious encephalomyelitis: Etiologic and diagnostic trends. Journal of Child Neurology 2000;15(10):666-670. DOI: 10.1177/088307380001501005. Erratum in: J Child Neurol 2000;15(12):802

[150] Cuadrado MJ, Khamashta MA, Ballesteros A, Godfrey T, Simon MJ, Hughes GR. Can neurologic manifestations of Hughes (antiphospholipid) syndrome be distinguished from multiple sclerosis? Analysis of 27 patients and review of the literature. Medicine (Baltimore). 2000;**79**(1):57-68. DOI: 10.1097/00005792-200001000-00006

[151] Dey AB, Trikha I, Banerjee M, Jain R, Nagarkar KM. Acute disseminated encephalomyelitis--another cause of post malaria cerebellar ataxia. The Journal of the Association of Physicians of India. 2001;**49**:756-758. Available from: https://pubmed.ncbi.nlm.nih.gov/11573566/

[152] Mohsen AH, McKendrick MW, Schmid ML, Green ST, Hadjivassiliou M, Romanowski C. Postmalaria neurological syndrome: A case of acute disseminated encephalomyelitis? Journal of Neurology, Neurosurgery, and Psychiatry. 2000;**68**(3):388-389. DOI: 10.1136/jnnp.68.3.388a

[153] Pohl D, Tenembaum S. Treatment of acute disseminated encephalomyelitis. Current Treatment Options in Neurology. 2012;**14**(3):264-275. DOI: 10.1007/s11940-012-0170-0

[154] Payne ET, Rutka JT, Ho TK, Halliday WC, Banwell BL. Treatment leading to dramatic recovery in acute hemorrhagic leukoencephalitis. Journal of Child Neurology. 2007;**22**(1):109-113. DOI: 10.1177/0883073807299971

Section 3

Management and Therapy

Chapter 5

Artificial Intelligence Algorithms in Neurology: Optimizing the Management of Patients with Multiple Sclerosis

Alexander Zakharov, Igor Shirolapov, Elena Khivintseva, Olga Pavlova, Natalia Romanchuk, Alexander Kolsanov, Mariya Sergeeva and Yulia Komarova

Abstract

Artificial intelligence (AI) and machine learning (ML) have revolutionized the field of neurology, particularly in the diagnosis and management of multiple sclerosis (MS). MS is a complex, immune-mediated neurological disorder characterized by demyelination and neurodegeneration, making early detection and continuous monitoring essential for effective treatment. Magnetic resonance imaging (MRI) is the gold standard for diagnosing MS, but traditional methods for lesion detection, segmentation, and disease progression assessment remain time-consuming and prone to variability. Recent advancements in AI-driven image analysis have significantly improved the accuracy and efficiency of MS diagnostics. Deep learning algorithms can automatically identify white matter lesions, quantify brain atrophy, and track disease progression with high precision. AI-powered models also enhance differential diagnosis by distinguishing MS from other demyelinating disorders, such as neuromyelitis optica spectrum disorder (NMOSD), through radiomics and multimodal data integration. Additionally, predictive AI algorithms analyzing MRI, cerebrospinal fluid biomarkers, and genetic data help forecast disease trajectories and treatment responses, enabling personalized therapeutic strategies. Despite these advancements, challenges remain in implementing AI for MS care, including data standardization, model interpretability, and ethical considerations related to bias and privacy. Explainable AI (XAI) and federated learning approaches are being explored to address these limitations and improve clinical adoption. The integration of AI with real-time patient monitoring tools, such as wearable sensors and digital biomarkers, holds promise for more comprehensive MS management. As AI continues to evolve, its role in neurology will expand, offering enhanced diagnostic accuracy, individualized treatment planning, and improved patient outcomes.

Keywords: artificial intelligence, multiple sclerosis, machine learning, MRI, neuroimaging, deep learning, personalized medicine

1. Introduction

Magnetic resonance imaging (MRI) represents one of the most groundbreaking advancements in medical diagnostics. Its origins can be traced back to the fundamental principles of nuclear magnetic resonance (NMR), a phenomenon first identified in the early twentieth century. Over time, these scientific discoveries evolved into a sophisticated imaging technique that has significantly enhanced our ability to study human anatomy and pathology.

The theoretical basis for MRI was established during the 1930s and 1940s through the pioneering work of physicists such as Isidor Isaac Rabi, Felix Bloch, and Edward Purcell. In 1938, Rabi demonstrated that atomic nuclei could be influenced by magnetic fields, an achievement that earned him the Nobel Prize in Physics in 1944. This method, referred to as molecular beam magnetic resonance, laid the groundwork for further advancements in the field [1]. In 1946, Bloch and Purcell independently discovered that nuclear spins absorb and emit radiofrequency energy when placed in a magnetic field. Their contributions were recognized with the Nobel Prize in Physics in 1952 [2].

Initially, these discoveries found applications primarily in chemistry and physics, particularly in molecular structure analysis. However, their potential for medical imaging was not fully explored until the early 1970s.

The transition from NMR as a research tool to a medical imaging technique was pioneered by Raymond Damadian, a physician and researcher. In 1971, he published a seminal study demonstrating that malignant and healthy tissues exhibit distinct NMR relaxation times, suggesting that this technology could be used to detect cancerous tissues [3]. Although early implementations of his method lacked the precision required for imaging, his research marked the beginning of the application of magnetic resonance in medicine.

At the same time, significant advancements in imaging techniques were made by Paul Lauterbur and Peter Mansfield. In 1973, Lauterbur introduced the concept of spatial encoding using magnetic field gradients, which enabled the generation of two-dimensional images [4]. Mansfield further refined this technique by developing echo-planar imaging, which dramatically improved both image acquisition speed and resolution [5]. Their pioneering contributions laid the foundation for modern MRI technology and were recognized with the Nobel Prize in Physiology or Medicine in 2003.

The construction of the first MRI scanners in the late 1970s marked a significant milestone in medical imaging. In 1977, Raymond Damadian and his team developed the first functional MRI machine, successfully producing a rudimentary image of a human chest. Shortly thereafter, prototypes designed by Paul Lauterbur and Peter Mansfield demonstrated vastly improved image quality, showcasing the potential of MRI as a powerful diagnostic tool. By the early 1980s, commercial MRI systems were introduced, revolutionizing clinical imaging. The formal integration of MRI into medical practice was solidified in 1984 with the U.S. Food and Drug Administration (FDA) approval of the first commercial MRI scanner.

The following decades witnessed rapid technological progress, significantly broadening MRI's clinical applications. Key innovations included:

- Gradient echo imaging, which facilitated faster image acquisition and enhanced flexibility in MRI protocols, improving the efficiency of diagnostic procedures.

- Functional MRI (fMRI), introduced in the early 1990s, which enabled the noninvasive visualization of brain activity by detecting fluctuations in blood oxygenation levels [6]. This breakthrough allowed neuroscientists to explore cognitive processes, sensory functions, and psychiatric disorders.

- Diffusion-weighted imaging (DWI) and diffusion tensor imaging (DTI), which enabled the study of white matter integrity and provided a critical tool for early stroke detection. DTI, in particular, allowed for the mapping of neuronal pathways, contributing to research on neurodegenerative diseases.

- High-field MRI systems, such as 3 Tesla (3 T) and later 7 Tesla (7 T) scanners, which provided significantly improved spatial resolution and contrast, allowing for more detailed visualization of fine anatomical structures.

These technological advancements firmly established MRI as an indispensable tool in both clinical practice and biomedical research. MRI's role expanded beyond diagnostics, enabling critical discoveries in neuroscience, oncology, and cardiology.

MRI has played a pivotal role in uncovering the structural and functional changes associated with numerous diseases. In neuroscience, advanced MRI techniques have provided crucial insights into neurodegenerative disorders such as Alzheimer's disease, Parkinson's disease, and multiple sclerosis (MS). Techniques like diffusion tensor imaging (DTI) and functional MRI (fMRI) have revealed disruptions in white matter integrity and functional brain networks, respectively, offering a deeper understanding of cognitive decline and motor dysfunction [7, 8].

For instance, in multiple sclerosis (MS), advanced MRI modalities such as T2-weighted imaging and magnetization transfer imaging have been instrumental in identifying demyelination and neuroaxonal damage, helping to elucidate both the inflammatory and degenerative aspects of the disease [9]. Similarly, in oncology, MRI has revolutionized tumor characterization by differentiating viable tumor tissue from necrotic regions using contrast-enhanced imaging and diffusion-weighted imaging (DWI). These techniques have significantly improved tumor grading, treatment planning, and response assessment, providing valuable prognostic information for patients [10].

As MRI technology continues to evolve, emerging innovations promise to further expand its capabilities. Ultra-high-field MRI ($\geq$7 T), artificial intelligence (AI)-assisted image analysis, and quantitative MRI techniques are poised to enhance both diagnostic precision and research applications. These advancements hold the potential to refine disease detection, improve early diagnosis, and personalize treatment strategies, further cementing MRI's role as an essential tool in modern medicine.

MRI's continued evolution has positioned it at the forefront of medical imaging, not only improving diagnostic accuracy but also paving the way for more personalized approaches to disease management. Emerging technologies are expanding MRI's capabilities, integrating artificial intelligence (AI), ultra-high-field imaging, and novel contrast agents to further refine diagnostic and prognostic assessments.

One of the most transformative developments in MRI is the integration of artificial intelligence and machine learning. AI-driven algorithms have demonstrated remarkable potential in automating image segmentation, enhancing image reconstruction, and improving diagnostic accuracy. Deep learning models can rapidly analyze large imaging datasets, detecting subtle patterns indicative of disease progression that may be imperceptible to the human eye [11]. AI-assisted MRI is particularly promising in neuroimaging, where it facilitates early detection of Alzheimer's disease and other neurodegenerative conditions by identifying structural and functional abnormalities before clinical symptoms manifest [12].

Ultra-high-field MRI, particularly at 7 Tesla (7 T) and beyond, is another frontier in advanced imaging. These high-field systems offer unparalleled spatial resolution, enabling visualization of microstructural changes in the brain, musculoskeletal system, and cardiovascular tissues with unprecedented detail [13]. In neurology, 7 T MRI has been instrumental in detecting cortical lesions in multiple sclerosis that were previously undetectable at lower field strengths, improving disease characterization and treatment planning [14]. Similarly, in oncology, high-field MRI enhances tumor delineation, aiding in more precise surgical and radiotherapy planning.

Advancements in contrast agents and molecular imaging have also enhanced MRI's diagnostic and therapeutic potential. Novel nanoparticle-based contrast agents and targeted molecular probes enable the visualization of specific cellular and molecular processes, allowing for early disease detection at the biochemical level [15]. In cancer imaging, for instance, molecular MRI techniques can differentiate between aggressive and indolent tumors by detecting biomarkers associated with tumor metabolism and micro-environment changes. Such approaches are transforming MRI from a purely anatomical imaging tool into a method for functional and molecular characterization of diseases.

Hybrid imaging modalities are further enhancing MRI's versatility. The combination of MRI with positron emission tomography (PET/MRI) is particularly impactful in oncology and neurology, allowing for simultaneous structural, functional, and metabolic assessments. PET/MRI has shown superior performance over PET/CT in detecting brain tumors, neurodegenerative diseases, and certain cancers, offering lower radiation exposure and improved soft-tissue contrast [16]. In cardiovascular imaging, PET/MRI is proving useful for assessing myocardial inflammation and fibrosis, contributing to more precise risk stratification in heart disease [17].

The future of MRI is also being shaped by its integration with multi-omics approaches, including genomics, proteomics, and metabolomics. By combining MRI-derived biomarkers with genetic and molecular data, researchers are uncovering new disease subtypes and identifying personalized therapeutic targets. In oncology, radiogenomics is emerging as a powerful field, linking imaging features with genetic mutations to predict tumor behavior and treatment response [10]. Similarly, in neurological disorders, multimodal imaging-genomic studies are shedding light on the genetic underpinnings of diseases such as Alzheimer's and Parkinson's, potentially leading to earlier and more targeted interventions [18].

As MRI continues to evolve, its role in precision medicine is becoming increasingly prominent. The integration of AI, high-field imaging, molecular diagnostics, and hybrid modalities is refining MRI's ability to provide individualized disease assessment and treatment planning. These innovations, combined with ongoing research into novel imaging biomarkers and personalized therapeutic strategies, are ensuring that MRI remains an essential tool in both clinical practice and biomedical research.

With its ability to bridge the gap between structural, functional, and molecular assessment, MRI stands at the intersection of cutting-edge technology and patient-centered care. Future advancements promise to enhance its diagnostic power, improve early disease detection, and support the development of novel therapeutics, solidifying MRI's role as a cornerstone of modern medicine.

2. Challenges in MRI-based diagnosis and monitoring of multiple sclerosis

Multiple sclerosis (MS) is a chronic, immune-mediated neurodegenerative disorder of the central nervous system (CNS) that results in inflammation, demyelination, and subsequent neuroaxonal damage [19]. Due to its extensive impact on the nervous system, MS presents with a highly heterogeneous clinical profile, making its diagnosis and monitoring particularly challenging [20]. Patients often experience a range of symptoms, including sensory disturbances (numbness, pain, or altered sensation), motor impairments (muscle weakness, spasticity, or coordination difficulties), autonomic dysfunction (bladder and bowel disturbances), visual disturbances, and cognitive decline. The severity and progression of disability in MS are typically assessed using the Expanded Disability Status Scale (EDSS), which remains a widely accepted measure in both clinical practice and research settings [20].

MS is classified into distinct subtypes based on its clinical course, including relapsing-remitting (RR), secondary-progressive (SP), primary-progressive (PP), and the less common recurrent-progressive (RP) forms. RRMS, which accounts for approximately 85% of cases, is characterized by episodic relapses—periods of acute neurological decline—followed by partial or complete recovery during remission phases [21]. Over time, a significant proportion of RRMS cases transition to SPMS, marked by a steady accumulation of disability with or without superimposed relapses, reflecting a shift toward irreversible neurodegeneration [21].

The accurate diagnosis and long-term monitoring of MS remain complex due to its heterogeneous clinical presentation, variable progression patterns, and the limitations of current diagnostic tools. Given the overlapping symptoms with other neurological disorders, including neuromyelitis optica spectrum disorder (NMOSD), small vessel ischemic disease, and systemic autoimmune conditions, the risk of misdiagnosis remains high [22]. Additionally, initial MS manifestations can be subtle or nonspecific, further complicating early detection. Patients may present with a variety of neurological deficits, including sensory disturbances, motor dysfunction, impaired coordination, and cognitive impairment, which can mimic other CNS pathologies [23]. This diagnostic uncertainty underscores the need for a multimodal approach that integrates clinical evaluation, neuroimaging, and laboratory biomarkers to enhance diagnostic accuracy and disease monitoring [24].

Magnetic resonance imaging (MRI) has become an indispensable tool in MS diagnosis and disease tracking, offering critical insights into structural and pathological changes in the CNS. As a noninvasive imaging modality, MRI detects variations in proton responses to radiofrequency pulses, allowing for the visualization of demyelinating lesions and neurodegeneration [19]. Standard MRI protocols for MS evaluation include T1-weighted, T2-weighted, and fluid-attenuated inversion recovery (FLAIR) sequences, which provide essential information on lesion burden, disease activity, and neurodegeneration. Among these, 3D-T1 imaging, with its isotropic resolution, enables more precise anatomical assessments by maintaining equal voxel dimensions in all directions.

Despite being the gold standard for MS imaging, MRI has inherent limitations. While it is highly sensitive in detecting white matter lesions, its specificity is suboptimal, as similar-appearing lesions may be found in other conditions such as migraines, aging-related microvascular pathology, and systemic autoimmune diseases [9]. This overlap complicates differential diagnosis and may lead to delays or inaccuracies in disease classification. Furthermore, conventional MRI sequences primarily focus on white matter abnormalities, whereas gray matter pathology—a key contributor to disease progression and cognitive dysfunction—often remains undetected using traditional imaging techniques [25]. The inability of standard MRI to capture gray matter damage limits its utility in fully characterizing MS pathology, highlighting the need for advanced imaging approaches that provide a more comprehensive assessment of both white and gray matter integrity.

Key pathological features of MS include the formation of demyelinating lesions and progressive neurodegeneration, leading to brain atrophy. Lesion burden, typically visualized on FLAIR and, to a lesser extent, on 3DT1 MRI scans, serves as an important predictor of progression to clinically definite MS [26]. However, accumulating evidence suggests that gray matter atrophy, particularly in deep gray matter and cortical regions, is more strongly associated with physical and cognitive disability in MS patients. A longitudinal study examining individuals with RRMS and SPMS over 4 years demonstrated that gray matter atrophy significantly contributes to neurological impairment, with distinct mechanisms driving atrophy in different disease subtypes [27]. Notably, gray matter loss may serve as a more reliable indicator of disability severity than lesion burden alone [28].

Accurately detecting gray matter atrophy and other neurodegenerative changes requires automated segmentation and labeling of brain structures in MRI scans. However, this process remains challenging due to the complexity of brain morphology and the need for high-precision analysis. Neuroimaging software such as FreeSurfer [29] and FSL [30] are widely utilized for brain segmentation and volumetric analysis. Despite their effectiveness, these tools frequently require extensive preprocessing steps, including image transformation and intensity normalization, to optimize accuracy. Additionally, manual review and correction are often necessary, particularly in clinical applications where segmentation errors can influence diagnostic decisions. The time-intensive nature of these analyses limits their routine clinical use, underscoring the need for more efficient automated methods.

Early identification of high-risk patients remains a major diagnostic challenge, particularly in cases of clinically isolated syndrome (CIS), the first neurological episode suggestive of MS [31]. Not all individuals with CIS progress to MS, making it essential to differentiate between those at low and high risk of conversion to clinically definite MS (CDMS). MRI biomarkers, such as lesion count and distribution, play a crucial role in stratifying risk; however, these markers alone are insufficient for definitive prognostication without integration with clinical and immunological data [26]. The presence of oligoclonal bands (OCBs) in cerebrospinal fluid (CSF) and specific genetic or serum biomarkers have been investigated as complementary indicators to improve risk assessment in CIS patients, though their predictive value remains under active study.

Monitoring disease progression in MS presents additional challenges, as conventional clinical assessment tools may not fully capture the multifaceted nature of the disease. The Expanded Disability Status Scale (EDSS) remains the most widely used measure of disability; however, it is primarily weighted toward mobility impairment and does not adequately reflect cognitive dysfunction or psychological symptoms, which are increasingly recognized as significant contributors to disease burden [32]. Furthermore, EDSS assessments are subject to inter-rater variability, and subtle changes in neurological function may go undetected in the early stages of disease progression.

MRI, the cornerstone of MS monitoring, provides critical insights into disease activity, but it has inherent limitations in tracking long-term neurodegenerative processes. While contrast-enhancing lesions and new or enlarging T2 lesions serve as markers of acute inflammation, they do not fully capture the underlying mechanisms driving long-term disability. Gray matter atrophy, which is increasingly recognized as a key predictor of cognitive decline and disability progression, remains challenging to quantify with conventional imaging techniques. Advanced neuroimaging methodologies such as voxel-based morphometry (VBM), cortical thickness analysis, and deep learning-based segmentation are being explored to improve the accuracy of gray matter atrophy assessment [9].

The growing recognition of gray matter pathology in MS has led to increased efforts to refine imaging protocols and develop novel biomarkers that better reflect disease progression. Techniques such as double inversion recovery (DIR) imaging, which enhances the visualization of cortical lesions, and ultra-high-field MRI (7 T), which improves the detection of microstructural changes, are being investigated as potential tools for earlier and more precise identification of neurodegenerative changes [25]. Additionally, emerging imaging modalities such as myelin-sensitive MRI techniques, including magnetization transfer imaging (MTI) and myelin water fraction (MWF) imaging, hold promise for assessing demyelination and remyelination dynamics in MS [33].

As neuroimaging technology continues to advance, integrating MRI findings with clinical, molecular, and genetic biomarkers will be critical for improving MS diagnosis and monitoring. The application of machine learning algorithms for automated lesion segmentation, atrophy quantification, and disease trajectory prediction is an area of active research, offering the potential to enhance the precision and efficiency of MS assessment. Future studies will need to address the translational challenges associated with these methodologies, ensuring their accessibility for routine clinical practice while maintaining robust validation in diverse patient populations.

Emerging imaging technologies and biomarkers continue to evolve, offering promising solutions to longstanding challenges in MS diagnosis and monitoring. Advanced MRI techniques such as double inversion recovery (DIR) and magnetization transfer imaging (MTI) are enhancing the detection of gray matter lesions and diffuse white matter injury, thereby providing a more comprehensive view of MS pathology. Additionally, quantitative susceptibility mapping (QSM) has gained attention for its ability to assess iron accumulation in deep gray matter, a process associated with neurodegeneration and disease progression [34]. Beyond imaging, fluid biomarkers such as neurofilament light chain (NfL) in blood and cerebrospinal fluid (CSF) have emerged as reliable indicators of axonal injury, reflecting disease activity and treatment response [35]. Elevated NfL levels have been correlated with acute inflammatory activity and long-term neurodegeneration, making them a valuable adjunct to imaging in tracking MS progression.

Despite these advances, integrating emerging technologies into routine clinical practice remains a significant hurdle. Many of these advanced imaging methods require specialized expertise, optimized acquisition protocols, and sophisticated post-processing techniques, which can limit their widespread adoption. Additionally, computational demands associated with high-resolution imaging and machine learning-based analyses pose logistical challenges, requiring substantial infrastructure and technical expertise. In resource-limited settings, financial constraints may further restrict access to these cutting-edge tools, necessitating the development of cost-effective and scalable solutions [36].

The complexity of MS necessitates a comprehensive, multimodal approach to diagnosis and disease monitoring. Combining clinical assessment with advanced imaging, fluid biomarkers, and computational tools may improve diagnostic specificity and better capture disease progression. Artificial intelligence (AI) and machine learning are increasingly being explored to address these challenges by automating lesion segmentation, quantifying brain atrophy, and integrating multimodal data for more precise disease characterization. AI-driven models have demonstrated potential in predicting disease trajectories, optimizing treatment strategies, and improving early detection of progressive disease stages. However, the successful translation of these technologies into clinical practice requires rigorous validation across diverse patient populations to ensure reliability, reproducibility, and clinical utility.

In summary, while substantial progress has been made in refining MS diagnosis and monitoring, several critical challenges persist. Enhancing diagnostic accuracy, improving methods for assessing neurodegeneration, and integrating novel technologies into routine clinical workflows remain key priorities. Future research should focus on developing standardized protocols, optimizing cost-effectiveness, and ensuring equitable access to advanced diagnostic tools. By addressing these gaps, ongoing innovations hold the potential to enable earlier detection, more precise disease tracking, and ultimately, improved clinical outcomes for individuals living with MS.

3. The rise of artificial intelligence in medical imaging

Ensuring the successful integration of AI into medical imaging also requires addressing regulatory, ethical, and practical considerations. Regulatory agencies, such as the U.S. Food and Drug Administration (FDA) and the European Medicines Agency (EMA), have implemented guidelines for the validation and approval of AI-driven medical technologies. However, the dynamic nature of AI models, which can evolve as they are exposed to new data, presents a challenge for traditional regulatory frameworks that rely on static validation processes [37]. Establishing continuous monitoring and adaptive validation protocols will be critical to maintaining the reliability and safety of AI systems in clinical practice.

Another key consideration is the integration of AI into existing clinical workflows. Many AI-driven imaging tools require substantial computational resources and expertise in data science, which may not be readily available in all healthcare settings. Furthermore, the adoption of AI in radiology and neuroimaging necessitates training programs for clinicians to interpret AI-generated outputs effectively. Implementing standardized AI interpretability guidelines and user-friendly interfaces can help bridge the gap between algorithmic insights and clinical decision-making, ultimately improving AI adoption in real-world settings [38].

AI-driven automation in imaging also raises ethical concerns related to patient privacy, data security, and algorithmic bias. Deep learning models rely on extensive medical datasets, often sourced from electronic health records (EHRs) and imaging archives. Ensuring robust data anonymization and encryption methods is essential to protect patient confidentiality and comply with regulations such as the General Data Protection Regulation (GDPR) and the Health Insurance Portability and Accountability Act (HIPAA) [39]. Additionally, mitigating bias in AI algorithms is a priority, as models trained on skewed datasets may produce inequitable outcomes across demographic groups. Strategies such as bias-aware training, federated learning, and diverse dataset curation can help improve the fairness and generalizability of AI applications in medical imaging [40].

Despite these challenges, AI's transformative potential in medical imaging continues to drive innovation, particularly in the field of multiple sclerosis (MS) research and diagnosis. In MS, AI-powered models have been instrumental in automating lesion segmentation, detecting subtle patterns of brain atrophy, and predicting disease progression with high accuracy. Studies have shown that AI can outperform traditional segmentation methods in identifying new and enlarging lesions, reducing intra- and inter-rater variability in lesion quantification [41]. Moreover, AI-based longitudinal analysis of MRI scans enables early detection of progressive changes in brain volume, offering a more sensitive marker of neurodegeneration compared to conventional clinical assessments [42].

AI is also enhancing precision medicine approaches in MS by integrating multimodal data sources, including MRI, fluid biomarkers, genetic profiles, and patient-reported outcomes. Machine learning algorithms can identify complex relationships between these variables, facilitating the development of personalized treatment strategies. For example, predictive models analyzing lesion dynamics and immunological markers have been used to assess treatment response and optimize therapeutic decisions for individual patients [9]. Such advancements hold promise for reducing treatment failure rates and minimizing unnecessary exposure to immunosuppressive therapies.

Looking ahead, the future of AI in medical imaging is likely to be shaped by advancements in explainable AI (XAI), federated learning, and real-time imaging analysis. XAI frameworks are becoming increasingly important for enhancing the interpretability of deep learning models, enabling clinicians to understand the rationale behind AI-generated predictions [43]. Federated learning, which allows AI models to be trained across multiple institutions without sharing raw patient data, is emerging as a viable solution for improving AI robustness while maintaining data privacy [44]. Additionally, real-time AI-assisted imaging analysis is being explored for applications such as intraoperative MRI, where immediate feedback on lesion characteristics could enhance surgical precision and patient outcomes.

In conclusion, AI is redefining the landscape of medical imaging, offering unprecedented opportunities for improving diagnostic accuracy, disease monitoring, and personalized treatment strategies. While challenges related to data quality, regulatory oversight, and ethical considerations remain, ongoing research and technological advancements continue to drive AI toward widespread clinical adoption. By integrating AI with multimodal data sources, developing explainable and fair AI models, and ensuring seamless clinical integration, the future of AI-powered medical imaging holds immense potential for transforming patient care and advancing our understanding of complex diseases such as multiple sclerosis.

4. Artificial intelligence in diagnosing multiple sclerosis

4.1 Automated detection and segmentation of lesions

Another significant limitation in AI-based lesion segmentation for multiple sclerosis (MS) is the interpretability of deep learning models. Many convolutional neural networks (CNNs) function as "black boxes," making it difficult to understand how they arrive at specific segmentation decisions. This lack of transparency poses challenges for clinical implementation, as radiologists and neurologists require confidence in AI-generated outputs to integrate them effectively into decision-making processes. Recent advancements in explainable AI (XAI) aim to address this issue by developing visualization techniques such as saliency maps and gradient-based attribution methods, which highlight the most relevant features contributing to model predictions [43].

Beyond segmentation, AI has also been instrumental in quantifying lesion evolution, an essential aspect of MS monitoring. AI-driven longitudinal analysis enables automated tracking of lesion changes over time, reducing the subjectivity associated with manual comparisons. Recurrent neural networks (RNNs) and long short-term memory (LSTM) networks have been explored for modeling temporal changes in lesion burden, allowing for more precise assessments of disease activity and treatment response (La Rosa et al., 2020). These approaches have the potential to improve early detection of disease progression, particularly in the transition from relapsing-remitting MS (RRMS) to secondary-progressive MS (SPMS), where subtle volumetric changes in lesions and brain atrophy precede clinical deterioration [42].

Moreover, AI-based approaches extend beyond lesion detection to assess brain atrophy, another key marker of MS progression. Cortical and subcortical atrophy measurements provide critical insights into neurodegeneration, which conventional MRI-based assessments often fail to capture adequately. AI-powered segmentation methods, such as those incorporated in FreeSurfer and DeepSurfer, enhance the precision of gray matter volume quantification, thereby offering a more comprehensive evaluation of disease burden [45]. Additionally, the combination of AI with advanced MRI techniques, such as susceptibility-weighted imaging (SWI) and quantitative susceptibility mapping (QSM), has facilitated the study of iron deposition in deep gray matter, a potential biomarker of neurodegeneration in MS [46].

Despite the progress in AI-based neuroimaging, translating these innovations into routine clinical practice requires addressing several technical and logistical challenges. The variability in MRI acquisition parameters across different institutions complicates the standardization of AI models, potentially affecting their performance when applied to unseen data. Harmonization techniques, such as domain adaptation and intensity normalization, are being explored to improve cross-center generalizability [47]. Additionally, federated learning—a decentralized AI training approach that enables models to learn from multi-institutional datasets without sharing patient data—has emerged as a promising strategy to enhance model robustness while preserving privacy (Sheller et al., 2020).

Furthermore, regulatory considerations play a crucial role in AI adoption for MS imaging. AI models used in clinical practice must undergo rigorous validation and approval by regulatory agencies such as the U.S. Food and Drug Administration (FDA) and the European Medicines Agency (EMA). The development of standardized evaluation benchmarks and prospective clinical trials will be essential to ensure the safety and efficacy of AI-assisted MS diagnosis and monitoring [48].

In conclusion, AI has revolutionized MS imaging by enhancing lesion segmentation, tracking disease progression, and improving neurodegeneration assessment. While challenges related to interpretability, generalizability, and regulatory approval remain, ongoing advancements in explainable AI, federated learning, and harmonized imaging protocols are poised to bridge these gaps. Future research should focus on integrating AI with multimodal data sources, including clinical, genetic, and fluid biomarker information, to develop comprehensive, personalized disease models. As AI continues to evolve, its role in MS diagnosis and monitoring is expected to expand, ultimately improving patient outcomes through more accurate, efficient, and individualized disease management.

4.2 AI-powered algorithms for differential diagnosis

Beyond lesion classification, AI has also been instrumental in analyzing microstructural changes in the brain, which can further aid in differentiating MS from other neurological disorders. Techniques such as radiomics and deep feature extraction allow AI models to quantify textural, morphological, and statistical properties of brain lesions that may not be visually discernible by radiologists [49]. These high-dimensional imaging biomarkers provide a more nuanced assessment of disease patterns, enhancing the precision of differential diagnosis. For instance, radiomic analysis has been used to distinguish MS lesions from ischemic white matter hyperintensities by identifying differences in lesion heterogeneity, shape, and distribution [42].

AI-driven multimodal integration has further improved diagnostic accuracy by combining MRI findings with clinical, laboratory, and genetic data. Multiple sclerosis, NMOSD, and other autoimmune demyelinating disorders often exhibit overlapping imaging features but differ in immunological markers, such as aquaporin-4 (AQP4) and myelin oligodendrocyte glycoprotein (MOG) antibodies [50, 51]. AI models trained on multimodal datasets can incorporate MRI, cerebrospinal fluid (CSF) biomarkers, and clinical parameters to generate probabilistic diagnoses, reducing diagnostic uncertainty [52]. Bayesian networks and ensemble learning techniques have been particularly effective in handling heterogeneous data sources, allowing for more comprehensive disease characterization [53].

The application of AI in spinal cord imaging has also been a significant advancement in MS differentiation. Spinal cord involvement is common in both MS and NMOSD, but lesion distribution patterns differ. While MS lesions are typically short, focal, and asymmetrical, NMOSD lesions tend to be longitudinally extensive, spanning three or more vertebral segments. AI-based segmentation and feature extraction methods have demonstrated high accuracy in identifying these patterns, enabling automated differentiation between these conditions [54]. Additionally, spinal cord atrophy, which is more pronounced in progressive MS subtypes, can be quantified using AI-assisted volumetric analysis, aiding in disease staging and prognosis assessment [55].

Despite these advancements, the clinical adoption of AI for differential diagnosis in MS faces several challenges. The availability of high-quality, annotated datasets is essential for training robust models, yet inter-center variability in MRI protocols and lesion annotation standards remains a barrier to widespread AI implementation. Efforts to establish standardized imaging repositories, such as the MSSEG dataset and the OASIS initiative, are crucial for improving AI model generalizability and reliability [56].

Another key challenge is model interpretability. Deep learning models, particularly CNNs, often operate as "black boxes," making it difficult for clinicians to understand how diagnostic decisions are made. Explainable AI (XAI) techniques, such as class activation mapping and attention mechanisms, are being developed to enhance model transparency by highlighting the most relevant features contributing to diagnostic predictions [43]. The integration of these interpretability tools into AI-assisted diagnostic workflows can improve clinician confidence and facilitate AI adoption in real-world settings.

Looking ahead, AI is poised to further transform differential diagnosis in MS through advancements in federated learning, real-time imaging analysis, and personalized diagnostic models. Federated learning, which allows AI models to be trained across multiple institutions without direct data sharing, holds promise for improving model robustness while preserving patient privacy. Real-time AI-assisted MRI interpretation could enable immediate differentiation between MS and other demyelinating disorders, reducing diagnostic delays and optimizing treatment initiation. Additionally, personalized AI models incorporating patient-specific imaging, clinical, and genetic profiles could refine disease classification and prognosis prediction, paving the way for more tailored therapeutic strategies [42].

In conclusion, AI has significantly enhanced differential diagnosis in MS by improving lesion classification, integrating multimodal data, and automating spinal cord imaging analysis. While challenges related to data standardization, interpretability, and clinical validation persist, ongoing advancements in AI methodologies and collaborative research initiatives are driving the field toward greater accuracy and clinical applicability. Future developments in AI-assisted diagnostics are expected to refine disease classification, reduce misdiagnosis rates, and ultimately improve outcomes for individuals with MS and related neurological disorders.

Efforts to improve AI-driven differential diagnosis in MS are increasingly focusing on enhancing model generalizability, interpretability, and fairness. One promising strategy is the implementation of federated learning, a decentralized approach that allows AI models to be trained across multiple institutions without directly sharing patient data. This method preserves privacy while enabling the development of more robust and diverse models capable of handling variations in imaging protocols and patient demographics [57]. Federated learning has already demonstrated success in oncology and neuroimaging applications, and its adoption in MS research could help mitigate biases associated with single-center datasets while improving the reliability of AI-driven diagnosis across different healthcare settings.

In parallel, advancements in explainable AI (XAI) are addressing concerns about the "black box" nature of deep learning models. Techniques such as saliency maps, Shapley Additive Explanations (SHAP), and Local Interpretable Model-Agnostic Explanations (LIME) provide transparency by visualizing which imaging features contribute most to a model's predictions [43]. In MS diagnostics, these methods can highlight lesion characteristics and anatomical regions that influence classification decisions, enabling radiologists to verify AI-generated outputs and increasing trust in automated systems. Moreover, hybrid AI approaches that combine deep learning with rule-based expert systems are being explored to further enhance interpretability, ensuring that AI decisions align with established diagnostic criteria [58].

Beyond model refinement, AI is playing an increasing role in predictive analytics for MS, extending beyond differential diagnosis to prognosis and treatment response prediction. AI models trained on multimodal datasets—including MRI scans, CSF biomarkers such as neurofilament light chain (NfL) and glial fibrillary acidic protein (GFAP), genetic markers, and clinical history—are being developed to forecast disease trajectories [42]. For example, machine learning algorithms analyzing lesion volume, brain atrophy rates, and inflammatory markers have demonstrated the ability to predict conversion from clinically isolated syndrome (CIS) to clinically definite MS (CDMS), as well as the likelihood of transition from relapsing-remitting MS (RRMS) to secondary progressive MS (SPMS). These predictive capabilities are critical for early therapeutic intervention, allowing clinicians to tailor treatment strategies based on an individual patient's risk profile.

AI is also being leveraged to optimize treatment selection and monitoring. Traditional methods for assessing disease activity, such as lesion load on MRI and clinical relapse rates, often fail to capture the full spectrum of neurodegenerative processes underlying MS progression. AI-driven analysis of longitudinal imaging data can identify subtle patterns of disease activity, such as microstructural changes in white and gray matter that precede overt clinical worsening. Additionally, reinforcement learning algorithms are being explored to recommend personalized treatment regimens based on patient-specific characteristics and real-time responses to therapy, potentially improving outcomes while minimizing side effects [59].

Despite these advancements, several challenges remain in implementing AI for MS diagnosis and management. Regulatory hurdles pose a significant barrier, as AI-based medical technologies require rigorous validation before being approved for clinical use. Agencies such as the FDA and EMA are developing frameworks to ensure AI models meet safety, efficacy, and ethical standards, but the dynamic nature of AI—where models evolve with new data—complicates traditional validation approaches [60]. Developing adaptive regulatory strategies that allow AI systems to undergo continuous learning while maintaining clinical reliability will be essential for widespread adoption.

Moreover, the ethical implications of AI-driven diagnostics warrant careful consideration. Bias in AI models, stemming from imbalanced training datasets, can lead to disparities in diagnostic accuracy across different patient populations. Studies have shown that underrepresented groups, including racial and ethnic minorities, may experience reduced AI performance due to limited data representation in training cohorts [40]. Addressing these disparities requires diverse dataset curation, bias-aware training algorithms, and ongoing performance audits to ensure equitable healthcare outcomes.

Looking ahead, the future of AI in MS diagnosis and management will likely be shaped by the integration of multi-omics data, wearable sensor technology, and real-time AI-assisted clinical decision support systems. Combining AI-driven imaging analysis with genomic, proteomic, and metabolomic profiles could enable deeper insights into disease mechanisms and facilitate the development of truly personalized treatment strategies [42]. Additionally, remote monitoring tools, such as AI-powered gait analysis from wearable devices and smartphone-based cognitive assessments, may complement MRI-based evaluations, providing a more comprehensive picture of disease activity in everyday life [61].

In conclusion, AI is transforming the landscape of MS diagnosis and differential diagnosis by enhancing imaging interpretation, integrating multimodal data, predicting disease trajectories, and optimizing treatment strategies. However, challenges related to model generalizability, regulatory approval, and ethical fairness must be addressed to ensure that AI benefits all patient populations equitably. By fostering collaborative research, regulatory innovation, and continuous validation, AI has the potential to revolutionize MS management, improving diagnostic accuracy, treatment personalization, and long-term patient outcomes.

4.3 Enhancing accuracy and efficiency with AI

The integration of AI into the diagnosis and monitoring of MS has not only improved lesion detection and brain structure analysis but has also expanded into predicting disease progression and optimizing treatment strategies. Predictive modeling using AI enables clinicians to anticipate disease trajectories, assess the risk of conversion from clinically isolated syndrome (CIS) to clinically definite MS (CDMS), and identify patients who are more likely to transition from relapsing-remitting MS (RRMS) to secondary progressive MS (SPMS). Machine learning algorithms trained on multimodal datasets, including MRI-derived features, clinical history, and cerebrospinal fluid (CSF) biomarkers, have demonstrated the ability to forecast long-term disability outcomes with high accuracy [42].

AI has also contributed to refining treatment response assessment by analyzing longitudinal imaging data and identifying subtle changes in brain structure that may indicate worsening disease activity. For example, deep learning models can detect microstructural alterations in white matter tracts and gray matter atrophy, which often precede clinical deterioration. These findings can help guide treatment adjustments, ensuring that patients receive timely interventions before irreversible damage occurs. Furthermore, AI-assisted analysis of treatment efficacy has been applied to drug trials, where automated lesion segmentation and volumetric measurements provide objective endpoints for evaluating new MS therapies [62].

Another area where AI has shown promise is in integrating imaging findings with fluid biomarkers and genetic data to develop personalized treatment approaches. For instance, AI models analyzing neurofilament light chain (NfL) levels alongside MRI features have been used to predict relapse risk and monitor neuroaxonal injury over time [63]. The combination of imaging and biomarker-driven AI models enables a more precise understanding of MS pathology and may contribute to the development of individualized therapeutic regimens tailored to a patient's specific disease profile.

In addition to its applications in clinical practice, AI is also enhancing MS research by enabling large-scale, data-driven discoveries. Natural language processing (NLP) techniques have been employed to extract relevant clinical information from electronic health records (EHRs), identifying patterns and risk factors associated with disease onset and progression [64]. This approach allows researchers to analyze vast amounts of patient data efficiently, uncovering new insights into disease mechanisms and treatment responses. Additionally, AI-driven harmonization techniques are being developed to standardize imaging data from multi-center studies, facilitating collaboration across institutions and improving the reproducibility of findings [56].

Despite these advancements, challenges remain in fully integrating AI into routine clinical workflows. One of the primary limitations is the need for large, high-quality, annotated datasets to train robust models. Many AI algorithms are developed using single-center datasets, which may not capture the diversity of imaging protocols, scanner types, and patient populations seen in real-world practice. Addressing this issue requires multi-center collaborations and the establishment of standardized imaging protocols to improve AI model generalizability.

Another challenge lies in ensuring that AI-driven diagnostic tools are interpretable and transparent to clinicians. While deep learning models have demonstrated remarkable accuracy, their decision-making processes often remain opaque, making it difficult for clinicians to trust AI-generated predictions. Explainable AI (XAI) techniques, such as gradient-weighted class activation mapping (Grad-CAM) and layer-wise relevance propagation, are being developed to improve model interpretability by highlighting the features that contribute to AI decisions [43]. These methods can help bridge the gap between AI outputs and clinical reasoning, facilitating greater acceptance and adoption of AI in MS diagnosis and management.

Ethical considerations are also central to AI deployment in MS care. Biases in training data can lead to disparities in diagnostic performance, potentially affecting certain patient populations disproportionately. For example, underrepresentation of certain ethnic groups in MRI datasets may result in AI models that are less accurate for those populations. Ensuring diversity in training data, developing bias-mitigation algorithms, and continuously auditing AI performance are essential steps toward achieving equitable AI applications in healthcare [40].

Looking ahead, future developments in AI for MS are likely to focus on the integration of real-time monitoring technologies, such as wearable sensors and digital biomarkers, with imaging-based assessments. AI-powered gait analysis, smartphone-based cognitive assessments, and remote monitoring of motor function could provide complementary data to MRI findings, offering a more comprehensive view of disease activity outside of clinical visits [59]. Additionally, advances in federated learning, which enables AI models to be trained across multiple institutions without sharing raw patient data, may improve model robustness while preserving patient privacy.

5. Conclusion

The integration of AI with radiomics and advanced MRI techniques has further expanded the potential of imaging in MS research and clinical management. Radiomics, which involves the extraction of quantitative imaging features such as texture, intensity, and shape descriptors, has provided a more nuanced understanding of lesion characteristics and brain tissue abnormalities. AI-driven radiomic analyses have been successfully applied to differentiate MS lesions from other white matter pathologies, such as small vessel disease, thereby improving diagnostic specificity [53]. Additionally, radiomics has enabled the identification of imaging biomarkers associated with disease progression, facilitating early detection of transitions from relapsing-remitting MS to secondary progressive MS [42].

AI is also being applied to multimodal data fusion, incorporating information from genetic, immunological, and biochemical biomarkers to refine MS classification and risk stratification. Recent studies have demonstrated that AI models trained on MRI scans, cerebrospinal fluid markers such as neurofilament light chain and peripheral blood profiles can improve the prediction of disease activity and treatment response. Machine learning techniques such as random forests and support vector machines have been employed to integrate these diverse datasets, uncovering complex relationships between molecular markers and imaging phenotypes. This multimodal approach is particularly promising for precision medicine, as it enables more tailored therapeutic strategies based on individual patient profiles.

A crucial development in AI-assisted MS research is the emergence of federated learning, a decentralized training paradigm that allows AI models to learn from data distributed across multiple institutions without requiring direct data sharing. Given the challenges of data heterogeneity and privacy concerns in medical imaging, federated learning has the potential to significantly enhance model robustness while maintaining patient confidentiality. By enabling AI models to train on diverse datasets from different MRI scanners, acquisition protocols, and demographic populations, federated learning improves the generalizability of AI algorithms and reduces bias in MS diagnosis and monitoring.

Despite these advancements, several challenges must be addressed before AI can be fully integrated into routine MS care. One major limitation is data standardization, as variations in MRI acquisition parameters and preprocessing methods can affect AI model performance. Efforts such as the MAGNIMS consortium and international imaging initiatives have been working toward developing standardized protocols to facilitate AI applications in MS (on behalf of the MAGNIMS study group) [65]. Ensuring that AI models are validated across multiple datasets and clinical settings is critical for achieving widespread adoption.

Another key challenge is the interpretability and transparency of AI models. Deep learning algorithms, particularly convolutional neural networks and transformer-based models, often operate as black boxes, making it difficult for clinicians to understand how decisions are made. Explainable AI techniques, such as saliency maps, Shapley Additive Explanations, and Grad-CAM, are being developed to enhance model transparency by visualizing the features that contribute to AI-driven predictions. Integrating these techniques into clinical workflows will be essential for ensuring trust and acceptance of AI-based decision support tools.

Ethical considerations also play a vital role in AI deployment for MS management. Biases in training datasets, particularly regarding demographic and ethnic diversity, can lead to disparities in diagnostic performance. AI models trained predominantly on data from Western populations may not generalize well to underrepresented groups, potentially exacerbating healthcare inequalities [40]. Addressing these issues requires the inclusion of diverse, representative datasets, ongoing model audits, and the development of fairness-aware AI algorithms.

Looking toward the future, AI in MS imaging is expected to expand beyond diagnosis and monitoring into real-time disease management. AI-powered wearable technologies, such as gait analysis sensors, digital biomarkers from smartphones, and remote cognitive assessments, may complement traditional MRI assessments by providing continuous, real-world data on patient function [61]. The integration of these digital health tools with AI-driven imaging analysis has the potential to offer a more holistic, patient-centered approach to MS care, allowing for early detection of disease activity and more timely therapeutic interventions.

In conclusion, AI has transformed MS imaging by improving lesion detection, refining multimodal disease characterization, enhancing prognostic modeling, and supporting precision medicine approaches. The continued development of AI-driven methodologies, coupled with improvements in explainability, data standardization, and ethical AI practices, will be crucial in realizing its full potential. As AI technology advances, its integration into routine clinical practice will likely optimize MS management, improve patient outcomes, and deepen our understanding of the disease's underlying mechanisms.

Conflict of interest

The authors declare no conflict of interest.

Author details

Alexander Zakharov*, Igor Shirolapov, Elena Khivintseva, Olga Pavlova,
Natalia Romanchuk, Alexander Kolsanov, Mariya Sergeeva and Yulia Komarova
Samara State Medical University, Russia

*Address all correspondence to: zakharov1977@mail.ru

References

[1] Rabi II. Space quantization in a gyrating magnetic field. Physics Review. 1937;**51**:652-654. DOI: 10.1103/PhysRev.51.652

[2] Bloch F. Nuclear induction. Physics Review. 1946;**70**:460-474. DOI: 10.1103/PhysRev.70.460

[3] Damadian R. Tumor detection by nuclear magnetic resonance. Science. 1971;**171**:1151-1153. DOI: 10.1126/science.171.3976.1151

[4] Lauterbur PC. Image formation by induced local interactions: Examples employing nuclear magnetic resonance. Nature. 1973;**242**:190-191. DOI: 10.1038/242190a0

[5] Mansfield P. Multi-planar image formation using NMR spin echoes. Journal of Physics C: Solid State Physics. 1977;**10**:L55-L58. DOI: 10.1088/0022-3719/10/3/004

[6] Ogawa S, Lee TM, Kay AR, Tank DW. Brain magnetic resonance imaging with contrast dependent on blood oxygenation. Proceedings of the National Academy of Sciences of the United States of America. 1990;**87**:9868-9872. DOI: 10.1073/pnas.87.24.9868

[7] Assaf Y, Pasternak O. Diffusion tensor imaging (DTI)-based white matter mapping in brain research: A review. Journal of Molecular Neuroscience. 2008;**34**:51-61. DOI: 10.1007/s12031-007-0029-0

[8] Frolov N, Pitsik E, Grubov V, Badarin A, Maksimenko V, Zakharov A, et al. Perceptual integration compensates for attention deficit in elderly during repetitive auditory-based sensorimotor task. Sensors. 2023;**23**:6420. DOI: 10.3390/s23146420

[9] Filippi M, Preziosa P, Banwell BL, Barkhof F, Ciccarelli O, De Stefano N, et al. Assessment of lesions on magnetic resonance imaging in multiple sclerosis: Practical guidelines. Brain. 2019;**142**:1858-1875. DOI: 10.1093/brain/awz144

[10] Aerts HJWL, Velazquez ER, Leijenaar RTH, Parmar C, Grossmann P, Carvalho S, et al. Correction: Corrigendum: Decoding tumour phenotype by noninvasive imaging using a quantitative radiomics approach. Nature Communications. 2014;**5**:4644. DOI: 10.1038/ncomms5644

[11] Lundervold AS, Lundervold A. An overview of deep learning in medical imaging focusing on MRI. Zeitschrift für Medizinische Physik. 2019;**29**:102-127. DOI: 10.1016/j.zemedi.2018.11.002

[12] Kumar R, Waisberg E, Ong J, Paladugu P, Amiri D, Saintyl J, et al. Artificial intelligence-based methodologies for early diagnostic precision and personalized therapeutic strategies in neuro-ophthalmic and neurodegenerative pathologies. Brain Sciences. 2024;**14**:1266. DOI: 10.3390/brainsci14121266

[13] Perera, Molligoda Arachchige AS, Politi LS. Potential applications of 7 tesla magnetic resonance imaging in paediatric neuroimaging: Feasibility and challenges. World Journal of Clinical Pediatrics. 2024;**13**(2):90641. DOI: 10.5409/wjcp.v13.i2.90641

[14] Abdel-Fahim R, Mistry N, Mougin O, Blazejewska A, Pitiot A, Retkute R, et al. Improved detection of focal

cortical lesions using 7T magnetisation transfer imaging in patients with multiple sclerosis. Multiple Sclerosis and Related Disorders. 2014;**3**:258-265. DOI: 10.1016/j.msard.2013.10.004

[15] Hellebust A, Richards-Kortum R. Advances in molecular imaging: Targeted optical contrast agents for cancer diagnostics. Nanomedicine. 2012;7:429-445. DOI: 10.2217/nnm.12.12

[16] Catalano OA, Masch WR, Catana C, Mahmood U, Sahani DV, Gee MS, et al. An overview of PET/MR, focused on clinical applications. Abdominal Radiology. 2017;**42**:631-644. DOI: 10.1007/s00261-016-0894-5

[17] Rischpler C, Nekolla SG, Heusch G, Umutlu L, Rassaf T, Heusch P, et al. Cardiac PET/MRI—An update. European Journal of Hybrid Imaging. 2019;**3**:2. DOI: 10.1186/s41824-018-0050-2

[18] Ciurea AV, Mohan AG, Covache-Busuioc R-A, Costin H-P, Glavan L-A, Corlatescu A-D, et al. Unraveling molecular and genetic insights into neurodegenerative diseases: Advances in understanding Alzheimer's, Parkinson's, and Huntington's diseases and amyotrophic lateral sclerosis. IJMS. 2023;**24**:10809. DOI: 10.3390/ijms241310809

[19] Dobson R, Giovannoni G. Multiple sclerosis – A review. European Journal of Neurology. 2019;**26**:27-40. DOI: 10.1111/ene.13819

[20] Kurtzke JF. Rating neurologic impairment in multiple sclerosis: An expanded disability status scale (EDSS). Neurology. 1983;**33**:1444-1444. DOI: 10.1212/WNL.33.11.1444

[21] McKay KA, Kwan V, Duggan T, Tremlett H. Risk factors associated with the onset of relapsing-remitting and primary progressive multiple sclerosis: A systematic review. BioMed Research International. 2015;**2015**:1-11. DOI: 10.1155/2015/817238

[22] Cree BAC, Arnold DL, Chataway J, Chitnis T, Fox RJ, Pozo Ramajo A, et al. Secondary progressive multiple sclerosis: New insights. Neurology. 2021;**97**:378-388. DOI: 10.1212/WNL.0000000000012323

[23] Zakharov AV, Vlasov IV, Poverennova IE, Khivintseva EV, Antipov OI. Posture disorders in patients with multiple sclerosis. Zhurnal Nevrologii i Psikhiatrii Imeni S.S. Korsakova. 2014;**114**:55-58

[24] Lezhnyova V, Davidyuk Y, Mullakhmetova A, Markelova M, Zakharov A, Khaiboullina S, et al. Analysis of herpesvirus infection and genome single nucleotide polymorphism risk factors in multiple sclerosis, Volga federal district, Russia. Frontiers in Immunology. 2022;**13**:1010605. DOI: 10.3389/fimmu.2022.1010605

[25] Geurts JJ, Calabrese M, Fisher E, Rudick RA. Measurement and clinical effect of grey matter pathology in multiple sclerosis. The Lancet Neurology. 2012;**11**:1082-1092. DOI: 10.1016/S1474-4422(12)70230-2

[26] Barkhof F. Comparison of MRI criteria at first presentation to predict conversion to clinically definite multiple sclerosis. Brain. 1997;**120**:2059-2069. DOI: 10.1093/brain/120.11.2059

[27] Fisher E, Lee J, Nakamura K, Rudick RA. Gray matter atrophy in multiple sclerosis: A longitudinal study. Annals of Neurology. 2008;**64**:255-265. DOI: 10.1002/ana.21436

[28] Fisniku LK, Chard DT, Jackson JS, Anderson VM, Altmann DR,

Miszkiel KA, et al. Gray matter atrophy is related to long-term disability in multiple sclerosis. Annals of Neurology. 2008;**64**:247-254. DOI: 10.1002/ana.21423

[29] Fischl B. FreeSurfer. NeuroImage. 2012;**62**:774-781. DOI: 10.1016/j.neuroimage.2012.01.021

[30] Jenkinson M, Beckmann CF, Behrens TEJ, Woolrich MW, Smith SM. FSL. NeuroImage. 2012;**62**:782-790. DOI: 10.1016/j.neuroimage.2011.09.015

[31] Zakharov AV, Khinivtseva EV, Poverennova IE, Gindullina EA, Vlasov IV, Sineok EV. Assessment of the risk of the transition of a monofocal clinically isolated syndrome to clinically definite multiple sclerosis. Zhurnal Nevrologii i Psikhiatrii Imeni S.S. Korsakova. 2013;**113**:28-31

[32] Cohen RA, Kessler HR, Fischer M. The extended disability status scale (EDSS) as a predictor of impairments of functional activities of daily living in multiple sclerosis. Journal of the Neurological Sciences. 1993;**115**:132-135. DOI: 10.1016/0022-510X(93)90215-K

[33] Moore BC. An Introduction to the Psychology of Hearing. Brill; 2012

[34] Quinn MP, Gati JS, Klassen ML, Lee DH, Kremenchutzky M, Menon RS. Increased deep gray matter iron is present in clinically isolated syndromes. Multiple Sclerosis and Related Disorders. 2014;**3**:194-202. DOI: 10.1016/j.msard.2013.06.017

[35] Zakharov AV, Bratchenko IA, Bratchenko LA, Neupokoeva AV, Khivintseva EV, Shirolapov IV, et al. Deep learning of surface-enhanced Raman spectroscopy data for multiple sclerosis diagnostics. The European Physical Journal Special Topics. 2025:1-9. DOI: 10.1140/epjs/s11734-024-01449-z

[36] Voigt I, Inojosa H, Dillenseger A, Haase R, Akgün K, Ziemssen T. Digital twins for multiple sclerosis. Frontiers in Immunology. 2021;**12**:669811. DOI: 10.3389/fimmu.2021.669811

[37] Hartung T, Kleinstreuer N. Challenges and opportunities for validation of AI-based new approach methods. ALTEX. 2025;**42**:3-21. DOI: 10.14573/altex.2412291

[38] Kelly CJ, Karthikesalingam A, Suleyman M, Corrado G, King D. Key challenges for delivering clinical impact with artificial intelligence. BMC Medicine. 2019;**17**:195. DOI: 10.1186/s12916-019-1426-2

[39] Alowais SA, Alghamdi SS, Alsuhebany N, Alqahtani T, Alshaya AI, Almohareb SN, et al. Revolutionizing healthcare: The role of artificial intelligence in clinical practice. BMC Medical Education. 2023;**23**:689. DOI: 10.1186/s12909-023-04698-z

[40] Mehrabi N, Morstatter F, Saxena N, Lerman K, Galstyan A. A survey on bias and fairness in machine learning. ACM Computing Surveys. 2022;**54**:1-35. DOI: 10.1145/3457607

[41] Valverde S, Cabezas M, Roura E, González-Villà S, Pareto D, Vilanova JC, et al. Improving automated multiple sclerosis lesion segmentation with a cascaded 3D convolutional neural network approach. NeuroImage. 2017;**155**:159-168. DOI: 10.1016/j.neuroimage.2017.04.034

[42] Eshaghi A, Young AL, Wijeratne PA, Prados F, Arnold DL, Narayanan S, et al. Identifying multiple sclerosis subtypes using unsupervised machine learning

and MRI data. Nature Communications. 2021;**12**:2078. DOI: 10.1038/s41467-021-22265-2

[43] Tjoa E, Guan C. A survey on explainable artificial intelligence (XAI): Toward medical XAI. IEEE Transactions on Neural Networks and Learning Systems. 2021;**32**:4793-4813. DOI: 10.1109/TNNLS.2020.3027314

[44] Rahman A, Hossain MS, Muhammad G, Kundu D, Debnath T, Rahman M, et al. Federated learning-based AI approaches in smart healthcare: Concepts, taxonomies, challenges and open issues. Cluster Computing. 2023;**26**:2271-2311. DOI: 10.1007/s10586-022-03658-4

[45] Yousef H, Malagurski Tortei B, Castiglione F. Predicting multiple sclerosis disease progression and outcomes with machine learning and MRI-based biomarkers: A review. Journal of Neurology. 2024;**271**:6543-6572. DOI: 10.1007/s00415-024-12651-3

[46] Zivadinov R, Tavazzi E, Bergsland N, Hagemeier J, Lin F, Dwyer MG, et al. Brain iron at quantitative MRI is associated with disability in multiple sclerosis. Radiology. 2018;**289**:487-496. DOI: 10.1148/radiol.2018180136

[47] Bashyam VM, Doshi J, Erus G, Srinivasan D, Abdulkadir A, Singh A, et al. Deep generative medical image harmonization for improving cross-site generalization in deep learning predictors. Magnetic Resonance Imaging. 2022;**55**:908-916. DOI: 10.1002/jmri.27908

[48] Han R, Acosta JN, Shakeri Z, Ioannidis JPA, Topol EJ, Rajpurkar P. Randomised controlled trials evaluating artificial intelligence in clinical practice: A scoping review. The Lancet Digital Health. 2024;**6**:e367-e373. DOI: 10.1016/S2589-7500(24)00047-5

[49] Zhang Y-P, Zhang X-Y, Cheng Y-T, Li B, Teng X-Z, Zhang J, et al. Artificial intelligence-driven radiomics study in cancer: The role of feature engineering and modeling. Military Medical Research. 2023;**10**:22. DOI: 10.1186/s40779-023-00458-8

[50] Shirolapov I, Zakharov A, Gochhait S, Pyatin V, Sergeeva M, Romanchuk N, et al. Aquaporin-4 as the main element of the glymphatic system for clearance of abnormal proteins and prevention of neurodegeneration: A review. WSEAS Transactions on Biology and Biomedicine. 2023;**20**:110-118. DOI: 10.37394/23208.2023.20.11

[51] Shirolapov IV, Zakharov AV, Smirnova DA, Lyamin AV, Gayduk AY. The significance of the glymphatic pathway in the relationship between the sleep-wake cycle and neurodegenerative diseases. S.S. Korsakov Journal of Neurology and Psychiatry. 2023;**123**(9):31-36. DOI: 10.17116/jnevro202312309131

[52] Kim A, Nigmatullina R, Zalyalova Z, Soshnikova N, Krasnov A, Vorobyeva N, et al. Upgraded methodology for the development of early diagnosis of Parkinson's disease based on searching blood markers in patients and experimental models. Molecular Neurobiology. 2019;**56**:3437-3450. DOI: 10.1007/s12035-018-1315-2

[53] Vrenken H, Jenkinson M, Pham DL, Guttmann CRG, Pareto D, Paardekooper M, et al. Opportunities for understanding MS mechanisms and progression With MRI using large-scale data sharing and artificial intelligence. Neurology. 2021;**97**:989-999. DOI: 10.1212/WNL.0000000000012884

[54] Vijendran M, Deng J, Chen S, Ho ESL, Shum HPH. Artificial intelligence for geometry-based feature

extraction, analysis and synthesis in artistic images: A survey. Artificial Intelligence Review. 2024;**58**:64. DOI: 10.1007/s10462-024-11051-3

[55] Liu Y, Dong D, Zhang L, Zang Y, Duan Y, Qiu X, et al. Radiomics in multiple sclerosis and neuromyelitis optica spectrum disorder. European Radiology. 2019;**29**:4670-4677. DOI: 10.1007/s00330-019-06026-w

[56] Commowick O, Combès B, Cervenansky F, Dojat M. Editorial: Automatic methods for multiple sclerosis new lesions detection and segmentation. Frontiers in Neuroscience. 2023;**17**:1176625. DOI: 10.3389/fnins.2023.1176625

[57] Sandhu SS, Gorji HT, Tavakolian P, Tavakolian K, Akhbardeh A. Medical imaging applications of federated learning. Diagnostics. 2023;**13**:3140. DOI: 10.3390/diagnostics13193140

[58] Zisad SN, Chowdhury E, Hossain MS, Islam RU, Andersson K. An Integrated Deep Learning and Belief Rule-Based Expert System for Visual Sentiment Analysis under Uncertainty. Algorithms. 2021;**14**(7):213. DOI: 10.3390/a14070213

[59] Hossain MZ, Daskalaki E, Brüstle A, Desborough J, Lueck CJ, Suominen H. The role of machine learning in developing non-magnetic resonance imaging based biomarkers for multiple sclerosis: A systematic review. BMC Medical Informatics and Decision Making. 2022;**22**:242. DOI: 10.1186/s12911-022-01985-5

[60] Mirakhori F, Niazi SK. Harnessing the AI/ML in drug and biological products discovery and development: The regulatory perspective. Pharmaceuticals. 2025;**18**:47. DOI: 10.3390/ph18010047

[61] University of California, San Francisco MS-EPIC Team, Cree BAC, Hollenbach JA, Bove R, Kirkish G, et al. Silent progression in disease activity–free relapsing multiple sclerosis. Annals of Neurology. 2019;**85**:653-666. DOI: 10.1002/ana.25463

[62] Krishnan AP, Song Z, Clayton D, Jia X, De Crespigny A, Carano RAD. Multi-arm U-Net with dense input and skip connectivity for T2 lesion segmentation in clinical trials of multiple sclerosis. Scientific Reports. 2023;**13**:4102. DOI: 10.1038/s41598-023-31207-5

[63] Bar-Or A, Thanei G-A, Harp C, Bernasconi C, Bonati U, Cross AH, et al. Blood neurofilament light levels predict non-relapsing progression following anti-CD20 therapy in relapsing and primary progressive multiple sclerosis: Findings from the ocrelizumab randomised, double-blind phase 3 clinical trials. EBioMedicine. 2023;**93**:104662. DOI: 10.1016/j.ebiom.2023.104662

[64] Zakharov A, Melnikova D, Shchepetov A, Andreev A, Dedyk D, Komarova Y. Automated MRI segmentation of patients with multiple sclerosis: Prospects for technology development. In: Sixth International Conference Neurotechnologies and Neurointerfaces (CNN). Kaliningrad, Russian Federation: IEEE; 2024, 2024. pp. 265-267. DOI: 10.1109/CNN63506.2024.10705810

[65] Wattjes MP, Ciccarelli O, Reich DS, Banwell B, De Stefano N, Enzinger C, et al. 2021 MAGNIMS–CMSC–NAIMS consensus recommendations on the use of MRI in patients with multiple sclerosis. The Lancet Neurology. 2021;**20**:653-670. DOI: 10.1016/S1474-4422(21)00095-8

Chapter 6

When and How to Use Plasma Exchange Therapy for Difficult-to-Treat Multiple Sclerosis Patients

Bhupendra O. Khatri and Jay S. Raval

Abstract

Therapeutic plasma exchange (PLEX) is a well-established therapy used for short- and long-term treatment of multiple sclerosis (MS), particularly for patients with steroid-refractory relapses and progressive disease subtypes. This chapter provides a comprehensive overview of the rationale, clinical evidence, and best practices for incorporating PLEX in the treatment of difficult-to-treat MS. It explores the mechanistic basis of PLEX in modulating immune responses and outlines predictors of clinical response, including MRI findings and timing of treatment initiation. Special attention is given to pediatric populations and the underrecognized value of long-term maintenance PLEX therapy in progressive MS. Practical guidance for vascular access, treatment protocols, and navigating insurance challenges is also presented to support clinicians specializing in care for MS patients who may benefit from PLEX.

Keywords: therapeutic plasma exchange, TPE, plasmapheresis, apheresis, PLEX, worsening multiple sclerosis, acute exacerbation, progressive multiple sclerosis, vascular access

1. Introduction

Therapeutic plasma exchange, also known as plasmapheresis or PLEX, is considered an immunomodulatory therapy as it helps modulate the immune system by removing harmful substances and inflammatory mediators from the blood. The removal of autoantibodies and immune complexes ensures a rapid onset of action, and the treatment is safe and effective for long-term use. Despite the fact that PLEX is widely used in the treatment of neurological diseases, its effectiveness has only been formally demonstrated in a limited number of conditions: myasthenia gravis (MG), Guillain-Barré syndrome (GBS), chronic inflammatory demyelinating polyradiculoneuropathy (CIDP), and multiple sclerosis (MS) [1–13]. While current disease-modifying therapies (DMTs) and especially high efficacy therapies (HET) are effective in reducing relapse frequency and inflammation, they are ineffective in treating a relapse, and 10–40% on HET do relapse [14]. While steroid treatment can help MS relapses improve faster, it is estimated that approximately 20–35% of patients may not fully respond to high-dose corticosteroids, meaning their symptoms persist or worsen despite treatment. PLEX is considered for steroid-refractory or severe relapses where steroids are ineffective or not tolerated. It removes potentially harmful substances from the blood, while steroids primarily target inflammation. A recent study found 73.8% of severe MS relapses showed marked clinical improvement after PLEX [15]. In a few relapsing MS patients with comorbidities such as prior or current malignancies, certain cardiac conditions, diabetic retinopathy, and immunocompromised status can preclude or restrict the use of these highly effective, immunosuppressive DMTs. There is also a primary unmet need in treating progressive forms of MS. This chapter will address when and how to use PLEX for these difficult-to-treat MS patients.

2. Pathophysiology and clinical course of MS

Understanding the pathophysiology of MS is crucial to understanding why PLEX is an effective therapy. MS is an immune-mediated disease of the central nervous system (CNS) and a leading cause of neurological disability in young adults in the United States. It is thought to stem from a failure of the body's immune system to select against autoreactive T cells and B cells. Autoreactive CD8+ T cells, CD4+ helper T cells, and TH17 cells that induce inflammatory responses in the CNS are thought to drive pathology. Autoreactive B cells also play a critical role as producers of cytokines that induce an inflammatory immune response via activation of autoreactive T cells. As such, higher levels of these autoreactive B cells are associated with an increased number of lesions and neurodegeneration as well as increased disability [16]. An interplay between cells that reside in the CNS, especially the microglia and hematopoietic cells that migrate into the CNS, cause the release of proinflammatory cytokines and inflammatory mediators resulting in chronic inflammatory process and leading to axonal loss and disability.

The most prevalent type of MS is relapsing-remitting MS (RRMS), which accounts for 80–85% of cases. RRMS involves periods of inflammation and damage to the protective coating of nerve fibers (demyelination), causing temporary acute worsening of symptoms (relapses) followed by recovery (remissions). An acute MS exacerbation typically lasts for at least 24 hours and occurs in the absence of other factors that could be causing the symptoms, often referred to as a relapse or attack. Over time, many people with RRMS progress to secondary progressive MS (SPMS), a stage of MS that follows an initial period of RRMS, characterized by a steady worsening of neurological function and increased disability, with or without occasional relapses or remission.

3. PLEX for MS and its mechanism of action

Understanding the mechanism of action of PLEX, which involves removing and replacing plasma, is crucial for explaining its efficacy in treating MS. Most DMTs for MS work by modulating the immune system, primarily by suppressing the activity of autoreactive immune cells that attack the myelin sheath in the CNS, thereby reducing inflammation and slowing disease progression. This is achieved through mechanisms like interfering with immune cell migration into the brain, altering the balance of T cell subsets, or directly depleting specific immune cell populations depending on the drug used. The immune-driven of MS makes PLEX a valuable treatment option. PLEX removes harmful proteins (like antibodies) from the blood plasma that are attacking the myelin sheath, while DMTs work to prevent the immune system from attacking the myelin sheath in the first place. By removing these proteins, PLEX aims to stop the attack on the myelin sheath and potentially reduce the severity and duration of MS relapses (flare-ups). Thus, PLEX is more effective in minimizing damage from an ongoing attack as opposed to preventing future attacks.

Since its first use as a therapy in the 1950's to treat hyperviscosity due to Waldenström macroglobulinemia [17], randomized controlled trials have demonstrated efficacy of PLEX in the treatment of a wide variety of diseases including thrombotic thrombocytopenic purpura (TTP) [18], acute inflammatory demyelinating polyneuropathy (AIDP) [19], MG [3], and CNS demyelination [20]. PLEX exerts its effects through multiple mechanisms of action [21]. It facilitates the removal of pathological antibodies and immune complexes from circulation, helping to reduce autoimmune activity. PLEX also eliminates pro-inflammatory cytokines and other inflammatory mediators that contribute to disease progression and can help redistribute antibodies from tissues and trigger immune system changes, providing benefits for people with demyelinating disorders. Furthermore, PLEX can restore regulatory immune cell populations, such as regulatory T cells (Tregs), and favorably modulate the balance between Th1 and Th2 helper T cell responses, contributing to a more regulated and homeostatic immune environment (**Figure 1**).

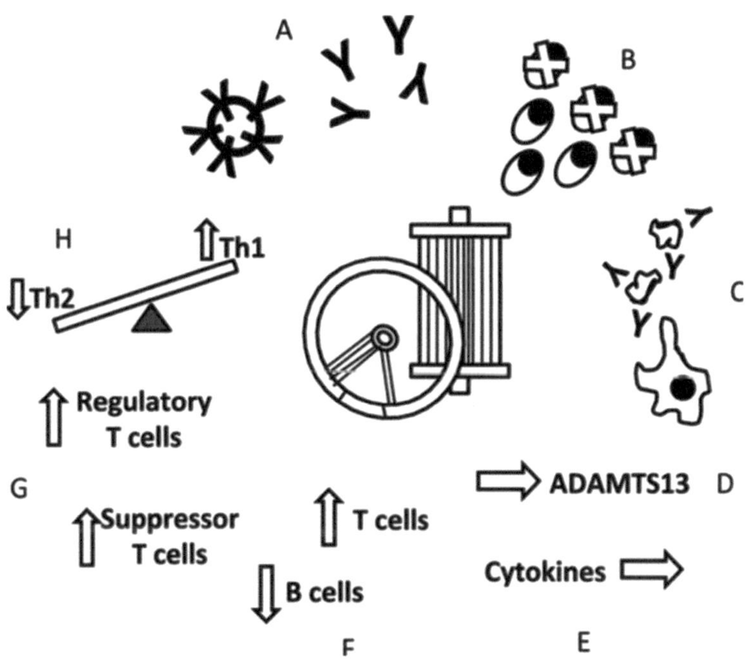

Figure 1.
Possible mechanisms of therapeutic plasma exchange. A. Removal of pathological antibodies. B. Stimulates the proliferation of B cells and plasma cells, sensitizing them to immunosuppressants. C. Removal of immune complexes with enhanced macrophage/monocyte function. D. Replacement of missing plasma components, such as ADAMTS13, a disintegrin and metalloprotease with thrombospondin type 1 motif, member 13. E. Removal of cytokines. F. Changes in lymphocyte numbers. G. Increased T regulatory cells and T suppressor activity. H. Correction of altered T-helper cell type 1/2. Courtesy of Jeffrey L. Winters, MD [21].

4. Role of PLEX in multiple forms of MS

In addition to its established role in acute, steroid-refractory cases, growing evidence supports the potential utility of PLEX in multiple forms of MS, especially when combined with immunosuppressive therapy. The following sections explore the current evidence base for PLEX in both acute and progressive MS, highlighting clinical outcomes, patient selection, and evolving treatment strategies. These and other related studies are summarized in **Table 1**.

Intravenous methylprednisolone, administered at doses of 500 to 1000 mg daily over 3 to 5 days, remains the standard first-line therapy for acute exacerbations of MS, owing to its ability to inhibit pro-inflammatory cytokine production, limit immune cell infiltration, and suppress broader inflammatory pathways. However, a substantial proportion of patients, estimated at 25–40%, fails to achieve meaningful recovery following corticosteroid treatment. In such steroid-refractory cases, escalation to PLEX is warranted.

PLEX is often effective for steroid-refractory relapses in MS, with studies showing improvements in a significant percentage of patients including those for whom standard high-dose corticosteroid therapy fails to control an MS relapse [15, 41]. Current guidelines recommend five to seven PLEX treatments administered over a 10- to 14-day period, with each session involving the exchange of 1 to 1.5 plasma volumes using albumin as the replacement fluid. In the most recent study [15], 73.8% of severe MS relapses showed marked clinical improvement after PLEX, 7.1% showed mild improvement, and 19.0% had no improvement. The median expanded disability status score (EDSS) significantly decreased from 6.0 indicating a high level of disability to 4.0 by the time patients were discharged from the clinic. This improvement was sustained at the six-month follow-up appointment. Based on these results, European and American guidelines consider patients with MS who have not responded to the treatment with intravenous pulse methylprednisolone as candidates for PLEX as a second-line therapy [42, 43].

Further support for PLEX as a second-line treatment for acute MS was provided by a double-blind, sham-controlled randomized trial evaluating the efficacy of PLEX in acute MS relapses. The investigators reported 42% of patients receiving true PLEX demonstrated moderate-to-marked functional improvement, compared with only 6% in the sham group [20]. Notably, differences became apparent as early as the third treatment session, supporting PLEX as a valuable rescue therapy for steroid-refractory exacerbations. Additionally, a North American muti-center, double-blind, randomized controlled study of 116 MS patients with an acute exacerbation measured the time to functional recovery using the Kurtzke EDSS [12]. All patients were treated with adrenocorticotropic hormone (ACTH) (40 U intramuscularly twice a day for 7 days, then 20 U twice a day for 4 days, and then 10 U twice a day for 3 days) and cyclophosphamide (2 mg/kg orally for 12 weeks), while half also received PLEX (1.5 plasma volume exchanges carried out five times in 2 weeks then every 6 weeks). The median time to recovery was significantly shorter in the PLEX-treated patients compared to sham-treated patients (4 versus 13 weeks). Additionally, EDSS scores remained increased by 0.79 in the sham-treated group at 3 months. This indicates that if PLEX is added to ACTH and cyclophosphamide to treat an acute attack, then the disability-recovery is *hastened* by 9 weeks. A PLEX protocol to treat an acute MS exacerbation is described in **Table 2**.

Study	N/ cohorts	Therapeutic Protocol	Results	Findings
Dau et al. [3]	8 Patients (1 Male 7 Females) Age range 33–51 yr. (Mean, 40.9 yr)	PLEX + Immunosuppression Protocol: • PLEX was conducted weekly or biweekly intervals; 50 mL plasma per kilogram of BW were exchanged each time. • Azathioprine, 2.5 mg per kilogram, was given at the onset of PLEX and continued during the follow-up period. • Prednisone, 100 mg daily, was given each morning for 4 days after each plasmapheresis.	• Modest improvement of neurologic function was reported; however, there was no change in auditory and visual evoked responses or serum demyelinating activity. • In 6/7 patients, cerebrospinal fluid IgG content decreased. • three additional patients in acute, severe exacerbation refractory to prednisone therapy made a substantial recovery, which commenced with plasmapheresis therapy. • In two of these patients the onset of clinical improvement after plasmapheresis was corroborated by decreased latency or increased amplitude of somatosensory evoked potentials.	PLEX protocol may afford modest benefit to progressive MS patients. Data are preliminary, and more research is necessary.
Tindall et al. [22]	20 Patients Overall *AZA:* 10 total (5 males, 5 females) Age 27–57 yr. (Mean 39.1 yr) *AZA + PLEX* 10 total (4 males, 6 females) Age 24–56 yr. (Mean 44.6 yr)	AZA Protocol: Patients received azathioprine 50 mg daily *AZA + PLEX* • Patients received azathioprine 50 mg daily increasing in 4 weeks to 3 mg per kilogram • Patients also underwent 3–4 plasma exchanges over 7 to 10 days; 5 to 6 liters with a total volume exchanged in the initial series of approximately six plasma volumes (one plasma volume = 5% of the body weight in kilograms). • A single two-plasma-volume • exchange was performed every 3 to 4 weeks for the next 12 months.	• No clear advantage was found for the PE + AZA treatment cohort compared with the group receiving AZA alone when looking at disability ratings • Five patients clearly progressed in the AZA group, and four patients clearly progressed in the PLEX + AZA group. • Of the patients who did improve, the most dramatic improvement occurred in the AZA group.	Plasma exchange and long-term immunosuppression offered no added benefit to long-term immunosuppression alone.

Study	N/ cohorts	Therapeutic Protocol	Results	Findings
		• Disability determinations • were done at 1 month, and at the same times as in the exchange group. At 12 months, evoked potentials, CSF, and laboratory investigations were repeated in both groups. • At 12 months, each therapeutic arm was compared, and progression was noted in each group.		
Hauser et al. [23]	58 patients overall *ACTH:* 20 total (8 males, 12 females) Ages at onset 29.2 ± 1.4 yr. Duration of chronic onset before study entry 2.1 ± 0.3 yr. *ACTH + CYCLO (Cyclophosphamide):* 20 total (7 males, 13 females) Ages at onset 25.4 ± 1.7 yr. Duration of chronic onset before study entry 2.9 ± 0.5 yr. *PLEX*: 18 total (9 males, 9 females) Age at onset 27.7 ± 1.2 yr. Duration of chronic onset before study entry 3.0 ± 0.6 yr	*Synthetic ACTH Protocol:* • Day 1–3: 25 U IV (8 h) • Day 4–6: 20 U IV (8 h) • Days 7–9: 15 U IV (8 h) • Day 10–12: 10 U IV (8 h) • Day 13–15: 5 U IV (8 h) • Day 16–18: 40 U IM Injection • Day 19–21: 20 U IM injection *ACTH + CYCLO Protocol:* • 10–14 Days (400–500 mg divided into 4 IV doses; 80–100 mg per kg of BW total dose per patient) • Treatment was discontinued if white-cell count fell below 4000/ cm^3 • Fluids (oral and IV) were administered to prevent bladder toxicity. • IV ACTH was administered via the protocol described above. *PLEX Protocol:* • PLEX was administered 4 or 5 times over 2 weeks. One to one and a half plasma volumes were removed per	• In the ACTH group, 8 of 20 patients at 6 months and 4 of 20 at 1 year stabilized or improved. • In the ACTH + CYCLO group, 18 of 20 at 6 months and 16 of 20 at 1 year stabilized or improved. • In the PLEX group, 11 of 18 at 6 months and 9 of 18 at 1 year stabilized or improved.	PLEX protocol was shown to have little impact on this drug regimen. Short-term, intensive immunosuppression (ACTH + CYCLO) was the most effective at halting progressive MS at 6 and 12 months.

DOI: http://dx.doi.org/10.5772/intechopen.1010410

Study	N/ cohorts	Therapeutic Protocol	Results	Findings
		• exchange and replaced with 5% serum albumin • All patients received ACTH as described for 21 days • All patients received oral cyclophosphamide (2 mg/ day) for 8 weeks and decreased if white-cell count fell below 4000/cm^3 Disability status score, ambulation index, functional-status score, and a quantitative neurologic examination were conducted prior to treatment, 6 months and 12 months post-treatment		
Gordon et al. [24]	20 patients total *PLEX:* 10 total (7 males, 3 females) Ages 28–47 yr. *Sham Exchange:* 10 total (7 males, 3 females) Ages 23–47 yr	• PLEX was administered three times weekly for 2 weeks, and twice in the 3rd week, for a total of 8 exchanges. One to one and a half plasma volumes were removed per exchange (1.5 h each) • Sham: total of 8 sham procedures (1.5 h each) • All patients received prednisone (30–50 mg every other day) and azathioprine (150 mg per day in three divided doses) begun at the onset of treatment.	• Assessments made post-treatment and 3–6 months later showed modest improvement in 7 of 10 patients in the PLEX group and 3 of 10 patients in the sham group. • Improvement was transient and there was no change in disability status scores.	This protocol for PLEX, combined with immunomodulating agents, are unlikely to be of clinical benefit to secondary progressive MS.
Khatri et al. [25]	45 patients total (13 males, 32 females) Ages 23–59 (mean 37.2) yr. Duration of MS before study entry 1–30 (mean 8) yr.	*PLEX + low level Immunosuppression Protocol:* • PLEX was administered weekly (1 PV exchange [5% of patient BW]) with replacement fluid of 5% albumin and normal saline for up to 10 exchanges and gradually longer intervals depending on patient's condition (until no further improvement was noted)	• 28 of the 45 patients improved significantly; 14 patients showed limited improvement; 3 patients neither improved nor worsened (as monitored by the Kurtzke Disability Status Scale [DSS] and functional systems scale, neuro-ophthalmologic evaluations, evoked	This protocol for PLEX, combined with low level immunosuppression, may offer improvement and stabilization in progressive MS, with minimal side effects.

Study	N/ cohorts	Therapeutic Protocol	Results	Findings
		• Low oral dose of cyclophosphamide (1 to 1.5 mg/kg of BW) daily and prednisone (1 mg/kg of BW) each alternate day in a gradually declining dosage was begun at the onset of PLEX and continued for one month after the last PLEX All patients were evaluated pre- and post-treatment and at 12 months.	potentials, computed tomographic scans, and suppressor cell function assays) • Significant improvement in suppressor cell function was noted in those patients whose conditions had improved by 1 or more steps on the DSS. • All but one patient required more than 10 PLEX treatments.	
Khatri et al. [10]	54 Patients Overall *PLEX + low-level Immunosuppression* 26 total (11 males, 15 females) Ages 36.3 ± 2.3 yr. Duration of MS before study entry 10.8 ± 7 yr. Duration of progression 2.1 ± 0.3 yr. *Sham + low-level Immunosuppression* 29 total (6 males, 23 females) Ages 42.2 ± 1.8 yr. Duration of MS before study entry 10.4 ± 1.0 yr. Duration of progression 2.7 ± 0.4 yr.	*PLEX + low level Immunosuppression Protocol:* • PLEX was administered weekly for 20 weeks (1 PV exchange [5% of patient BW]) with replacement fluid of 5% albumin and normal saline • Low oral dose of cyclophosphamide (1.5 mg/kg of BW) daily and prednisone (1 mg/kg of BW) each alternate day in a gradually declining dosage after week 15. This was initiated at the onset of PLEX and continued for 21 weeks) *Sham + low level Immunosuppression Protocol:* • Sham plasma exchange (patients received their own plasma as replacement fluid) was conducted weekly for 20 weeks • Low-dose immunosuppression was carried out as described earlier In addition, all patients received pooled human immune serum globulin-a total of 40 mL in four divided IM injections over 2 days after each PLEX or sham procedure.	• 14/ 26 patients who received PLEX and low-level immunosuppression demonstrated improvement (1 one step in DSS; mean change of 2.6); 11 were stable. Changes were sustained in 23/26 patients at follow-up. • For patients receiving low-level immunosuppression alone, improvement was observed in 8 (2 one step in Kurtzke DSS, mean change of 1.5) with stabilization seen in 11 patients. Changes were sustained in 23 patients at follow up. • Differences in improvement of PLEX + low-level immunosuppression over and sham + low level immunosuppression were significant at $p < 0.007$.	This protocol for PLEX, combined with low level immunosuppression, may offer improvement and stabilization in progressive MS, with minimal side effects (and afford greater benefit than immunosuppression alone).

Study	N/ cohorts	Therapeutic Protocol	Results	Findings
The Canadian Cooperative Group [26]	168 patients overall *Prednisone + Cyclophosphamide:* 55 total (18 males, 37 females) Ages at onset 31.9 ± 10.3 yr. Duration of MS before study entry 9.2 ± 6.4 yr. *Prednisone + Cyclophosphamide + PLEX:* 57 total (24 males, 33 females) Ages at onset 29.9 ± 7.9 yr. Duration of MS before study entry 9.4 ± 5.4 yr. *Placebo / Sham:* 56 total (24 males, 32 females) Ages at onset 32.1 ± 9.7 yr. Duration of MS before study entry 10.4 ± 6.7 yr.	*Prednisone + Cyclophosphamide Protocol:* • IV cyclophosphamide (1 g alternate days) and oral prednisone (40 mg orally for 10 days • The dose was reduced by 10 mg on alternate days and prednisone discontinued on day 16) *Prednisone + Cyclophosphamide + PLEX Protocol:* • Daily oral cyclophosphamide (1.5–2.0 mg/kg), alternate day prednisone (20 mg tapered) over 22 weeks. • PLEX 1 PV (40 mL/ kg) was exchanged weekly for 20 weeks (replacement fluid 5% serum albumin) *Placebo / Sham Protocol:* • Placebo medications (same regimen of administration as above) for 22 weeks • Sham plasma exchange (patients received their own plasma as replacement fluid) for 20 weeks All patients were followed for at least 12 months (mean duration of study 30.4 months with assessments every 6 months)	• No significant differences among the treatment groups for the primary analysis which comprised a comparison of rates of treatment failure. • No differences in the proportions improved, stabilized, or worsened at each 6-month assessment or in the mean change in the EDSS at the final assessment. • Slight positive trend the plasma exchange group at 12–24 months of follow-up was not sustained at the final assessment.	• No significant difference in outcomes compared to sham-controls. • Results were confounded by frequent and uncontrolled use of corticosteroid in patients who clinically worsened; these patients were not classified as "treatment failure". • Further analysis that controlled for corticosteroid use confirmed PLEX delayed the time to treatment failure.
Vamvakas et al. [27]	Meta-analysis 6 studies were evaluated Those reported in this table include: Khatri et al. [10] Canadian Cooperative group et al. [26] Hauser et al. [23] Gordon et al. [24] Tindall et al. [22]	Three outcome measures were studied: • The change in Kurtzke's disability status scale (DSS) scores • The relative odds of neurologic decline by 1 or more DSS grades • The relative odds of • neurologic improvement by 1 or more DSS grades, in the treatment versus the comparison group of patients.	The application of PLEX significantly ($P < 0.05$) reduced the proportion of patients who experienced neurologic decline (by 1 or more DSS grades) at 12 months of follow-up (relative odds of decline = 0.441, 95% confidence interval = 0.21 N.929).	There is benefit to the application of PLEX for chronic progressive MS. This must be explored further and may involve identifying and targeting specific subgroups within the chronic progressive MS patient pool who might respond best.

Study	N/ cohorts	Therapeutic Protocol	Results	Findings
		Reported results of neurologic evaluations at 6, 12, 24, and 36 months of follow-up were analyzed separately.		
Linker et al. [28]	2 Case Studies *Case 1:* 52 year old female with progressive MS with superimposed relapses for 40 months. Despite glatiramer acetate treatment, both leg palsy progresses and EDSS increased. The patient required bilateral aid for walking. *Case 2:* 49 year old female with 30-year history of MS; progressive MS for 10 years with superimposed relapses under treatment with interferon beta, mitoxantrone, and 3 months MP pulses. She was ambulatory with bilateral aid and EDSS 6.5.	*Case 1:* 5 weeks after the presentation of symptoms (unresponsive to MP) underwent 5 cycles of PLEX (50 mL/kg BW, replacement fluid albumin). *Case 2:* Before admission the patient suffered another relapse and required a wheelchair (EDSS 7.0) (Unresponsive to MP) 5 weeks after the presentation of symptoms the patient underwent 5 cycles of PLEX (50 mL/ kg BW, replacement fluid albumin).	*Case 1:* After 3 cycles there was significant improvement in right leg strength and by 5 cycles the patient was walking with only unilateral assistance (40 m) (and was further treated with mitoxantrone). *Case 2:* After 4 cycles there was significant improvement and on discharge the patient was able to walk with bilateral aid (30 m) (EDSS 6.5) (and was further treated with 3 monthly MP pulses)	While these are only 2 cases studies, the PLEX protocol employed may be most relevant and afford benefit to superimposed relapses in chronic progressive MS (although the durability of improvement was not shown in these cases).
Grapsa et al. [29]	10 patients total (7 males, 3 females) Ages 27–53 yr.	*PLEX Protocol:* • PLEX was administered three times a week for two weeks, followed by once weekly or monthly sessions based on stability. • Patients received PLEX combined with immunomodulating agents (interferon, azathioprine, or glatiramer acetate) for 18 months, then PLEX alone for an additional 18 months.	• After 36 months, five patients showed stabilization of disability, two experienced minor progression (0.5 EDSS point), and no relapses occurred • Spasticity improved in all patients (one experienced remission of cerebellar tremor) • At baseline, all patients showed enhancing lesions. • By the end of the study, seven patients had no enhancing lesions (with two developing more T2 lesions).	This protocol for PLEX, combined with immunomodulating agents, may offer stabilization and symptom relief in secondary progressive MS, with minimal side effects.

Study	N/ cohorts	Therapeutic Protocol	Results	Findings
Magaña et al. [30]	153 patients with steroid-refractory CNS-IDD treated with PLEX (1990–2007) (49 males, 104 females). Median age: 44 years (range 6–76). Most common diagnoses: Multiple sclerosis (MS): 48% Longitudinally extensive transverse myelitis (LETM): 24% Neuromyelitis potica (NMO): 17%.	• PLEX was administered as a rescue therapy for CNS-IDD attacks refractory to steroids. • Median of 7 exchanges (range: 2–24). • PLEX was initiated 23 days (median) after index attack.	• 59% of patients exhibited moderate-to-marked functional improvement within 6 months. • Response rates by diagnosis: LETM: 69%, MS: 62%, NMO: 42%. • Patients with shorter disease duration at PLEX initiation had higher response rates (median 1.1 years for responders vs. 2.3 years for non-responders). • MRI findings of ring-enhancing lesions or mass effect were strongly predictive of PLEX response (OR = 4.0 for RELs). • Preserved deep tendon reflexes associated with higher response rates. • Early initiation of PLEX correlated with better outcomes but benefit observed even beyond 90 days from attack onset.	• Findings support a humoral immunopathogenesis in some CNS-IDD cases, including MS (Immunopattern II) and NMO. • Results are consistent with PLEX as an effective option in steroid-refractory cases, though responses are variable and may depend on pathology.
Weinshenker et al. [20]	22 patients with acute MS attacks treated with true (n = 11) or sham (n = 11) PLEX. Age: Median 38 years (range 18–62).	• Double-blind, sham-controlled trial. • Patients were randomized to receive true PLEX or sham PLEX (control) over 7 treatments in 14 days. • All patients were concurrently treated with immunosuppressive therapies, including corticosteroids.	42% of patients in the true PLEX group showed moderate-to-marked functional improvement compared to 6% in the sham group. Significant differences in outcomes emerged by the third exchange. True PLEX led to better recovery of motor and sensory functions. No serious adverse events directly attributable to PLEX.	• PLEX demonstrated clear efficacy as an adjunct therapy in steroid-refractory acute MS attacks. • Early response predicts overall success. • Study supports the hypothesis that humoral factors contribute to neurological deficits in acute MS attacks, and their removal via PLEX is beneficial.
Rolfes et al. [31]	Systematic review of 63 studies on PLEX and immunoadsorption (IA) for acute MS relapses. Studies include: 63 publications, evaluating patients with RRMS, CIS, NMO, ON.	PLEX: 4–7 sessions, 0.6–2.5 plasma volumes per session. IA: Selective adsorption of immunoglobulins (IgG/IgM) using tryptophan-based adsorbers.	• PLEX response rates: 42–90% marked to moderate improvement. • IA response rates: 50–86% marked to moderate improvement.	• PLEX and IA are equally effective for treating steroid-refractory acute MS relapses.

Study	N/ cohorts	Therapeutic Protocol	Results	Findings
		Both methods studied post-steroid failure.	• Predictors: Shorter disease duration and early apheresis initiation improve response. • Functional improvements typically seen after 3–5 cycles.	• IA showed lower rates of adverse effects compared to PLEX (e.g., hypotension, infection). • Early initiation (≤6 weeks post-symptom onset) maximizes efficacy. • Guidelines recommend PLEX as first-line apheresis in MS relapses but acknowledge IA as an alternative with comparable efficacy and improved safety.
Ehler et al. [32]	37 patients with GCS-unresponsive MS relapses. Cohort: 6 CIS, 24 RRMS, 6 SPMS, 1 PPMS. Age: Median 32 years (15–73).	GCS (Relapse A): 1 g methylprednisolone (MP) daily for 5 days; in 48.7%, an additional 2 g MP daily for severe cases. PLEX (Relapse A): 3–9 sessions (median 5). GCS (Relapse B): Retreatment with 1–2 g MP daily for new relapse post-PLEX.	• Relapse A (GCS-only): No marked improvement. Moderate improvement in 5/37 (13.5%). • Relapse A (PLEX): Marked improvement in 32% and moderate improvement in 48%. • Relapse B (GCS after PLEX): Marked improvement in 27%, moderate in 65%. • EDSS scores improved significantly post-PLEX and relapse B GCS.	• PLEX is effective in GCS-unresponsive MS relapses, showing marked to moderate improvement in 81%. • Patients regain GCS-responsiveness after PLEX, favoring its use in subsequent relapses. • EDSS and clinical outcomes highlight humoral-mediated neuroinflammation as a potential treatment target in MS. • Study supports GCS as first-line for relapses, with PLEX for severe unresponsive cases.
Lehmann et al. [33]	Summary of studies on PLEX in MS and other inflammatory CNS disorders. Included conditions: MS (chronic progressive, acute exacerbations), NMO, ADEM, Rasmussen's encephalitis.	• PLEX: 5–11 treatment cycles, 1–1.5 plasma volumes exchanged per session. Replacement fluids: Albumin and/or saline, or fresh-frozen plasma (specific cases). • Combined with immunosuppression (e.g., prednisone, cyclophosphamide).	• PLEX improved clinical outcomes in acute exacerbations of MS and other CNS demyelinating conditions. • Response rate in acute MS relapses: 42–72%. • Limited efficacy in chronic progressive MS. • Beneficial in NMO with antibody-mediated lesions, particularly in Pattern II pathology.	• PLEX is most effective for steroid-refractory acute CNS demyelinating attacks. • It works by removing autoantibodies, complement components, and cytokines. • Best outcomes observed when combined with immunosuppression.

Study	N/ cohorts	Therapeutic Protocol	Results	Findings
				• Adverse effects: Hypocalcemia, infections, venous thrombosis, and hypotension reported but generally mild. • Early PLEX initiation correlates with better outcomes.
Correia et al. [34]	46 patients with severe steroid-refractory MS relapses. 84.8% RRMS (n = 39), 15.2% SPMS (n = 7). Mean age: 38.8 years; 76.1% female.	• PLEX: Mean 7.39 sessions (range 1–14), initiated after high-dose IV methylprednisolone (1 g/day for 6.1 days). Timing: PLEX started on average 33.5 days post-relapse onset. • Replacement fluids: Albumin or saline.	• Clinical improvement: 80.4% showed recovery; complete EDSS recovery in 41.3% and partial recovery in 39.1%. • MRI: Gadolinium-enhancing lesions in 68.8% of cases (n = 22). • Mean EDSS decrease: Median reduced from 4.0 (relapse) to 2.75 post-PLEX.	• PLEX effective for severe MS relapses unresponsive to steroids. • Early initiation enhances outcomes, but recovery observed even when delayed. • Higher sessions (≥9) associated with greater recovery. • Safety: 89.1% with no adverse events. Reported events included mild anemia, hypoalbuminemia, DVT, and transient hypotension.
Keegan et al. [35]	59 patients with severe CNS demyelination (RRMS, NMO, ADEM). 37.3% RRMS (n = 22), 16.9% NMO (n = 10), 16.9% ADEM (n = 10). Mean age: 41.4 years; 63% female.	• PLEX: Median 7 sessions (range 2–20) exchanging 1.1–1.4 plasma volumes. • Replacement fluids: Albumin (70%) or fresh frozen plasma. • Adjunct therapies: Prior high-dose corticosteroids (92%), immunosuppressants in some cases.	• Clinical improvement: 44.1% with moderate/marked improvement. • Response rates: 60% in NMO, 40% in RRMS. • Early responders improved within 3 PE sessions. • EDSS reduction: Median initial EDSS = 8.0; significant improvement in responsive patients. • 42.4% showed no improvement.	• Predictors of response: Male sex, preserved reflexes, and early initiation (≤20 days from onset). • Pathology-specific effects: Greater efficacy in humoral-dominant pathology (e.g., NMO). • Safety: PE well-tolerated; complications in 16.9% (e.g., hypotension, anemia). • Study highlights variability in response based on demyelination mechanisms and timing of intervention.

Study	N/ cohorts	Therapeutic Protocol	Results	Findings
Ehler et al. [36]	90 patients (28 males, 62 females): 46 RRMS, 21 CIS, 18 SPMS, 5 PPMS. Age: Median 38 years (range 18–69).	• PLEX Protocol: 5 sessions (median), max 8. Plasma volume exchanged: 2.8 L/session. • Replacement fluids: Albumin or Ringer lactate (5%). • Patients had prior high-dose IV GCS treatment (67.9%).	• Response rate: 72.2% overall. Marked improvement in 20%, moderate in 52.2%. • Relapsing forms (CIS, RR-MS): Response rate 81–82.6%. • Progressive forms (SPMS, PPMS): Response rate 38.9–60%. • EDSS decreased from 3.75 (baseline) to 3.0 post-PLEX.	• Relapsing diseases (CIS, RRMS) respond better than progressive forms (SPMS, PPMS). • Gadolinium-enhancing lesions on MRI were the strongest predictor of positive response. • Time to PLEX (median: 57.5 days) did not strongly affect outcomes.
Korkmaz et al. [37]	260 patients (130 males, 130 females) with autoimmune neurological diseases (45.4%, 26.1% MG, 19.2% MS, 1.9% PNS, 1.5% CIDP, 1.2% MOGAD). Median age: 50 years (range: 18–87)	• PLEX: Median 5 sessions (range 1–11). • Replacement fluids: 80% albumin, 17.7% FFP, 2.3% combination. • Vascular access: 99.6% CVC.	• Response rates: 21.7% CR, 59.6% partial (PR), 17.3% no response (NR). • Disease-specific outcomes: GBS: 80.5% response, MG: 77.1% response, MS: 94% response. • Adverse events: 12.7% (e.g., allergic reactions, catheter issues).	• PLEX is effective and safe for autoimmune neurological diseases, particularly in steroid-refractory cases. • Higher efficacy in conditions like MS and GBS; progressive diseases show lower response rates. • Early initiation improves GBS outcomes; safety profile is favorable.
Bunganic et al. [38]	155 RRMS patients (with severe, steroid-refractory relapses. Median age: 41 years (IQR: 33–47); 74% female. Exclusion: Progressive forms, prior PLEX.	• PLEX Protocol: 3–5 PLEX sessions performed every other day. • Plasma volume exchanged: 1.0 per session using albumin (67%) and saline replacement fluids. • Prior IV methylprednisolone (85%) or PLEX alone (15%).	• Response rate: 50% showed EDSS improvement; 37% remained unchanged; 13% worsened. • Median baseline EDSS = 4.5 (IQR 3.5–5.5). • Significant EDSS reduction observed after PLEX ($p < 0.001$). • No sex-based difference except slight favor for females ($p = 0.048$).	• PE led to significant improvement in severe steroid-refractory demyelinating attacks • Early PE initiation (<15 days) and clinical improvement at discharge were strong predictors of sustained response at 6 months (OR 6.29 and 7.32, respectively) • Non-MS patients responded better than MS, though not statistically significant in adjusted analysis • 48% of those not improved at discharge showed delayed benefit

Study	N/ cohorts	Therapeutic Protocol	Results	Findings
				• PE was well-tolerated; adverse events were manageable and mostly related to catheter use • Authors recommend not excluding late PE candidates (>60 days), as some still improved
Blechinger et al. [39]	118 patients with steroid-refractory MS relapses. Median age: 37 years (range 15–73); 64.4% female. RMS (83.1%) and PMS (16.9%)	• PLEX: 3–7 sessions. • Performed after IV methylprednisolone (15 g median total dose). • Replacement fluids: Albumin or saline.	• Response rate: 78.8% improved (43.2% marked, 35.6% mild); 21.2% no response. • Better outcomes in RMS (90.2% improvement) compared to PMS (64%). • EDSS improved by median of 1.0 point.	• Predictors of response: younger age, RMS diagnosis, gadolinium-enhancement on MRI, and early PLEX initiation. • Delay in PLEX initiation reduces response likelihood (7-day delay decreases response by 30%). • Safe and well-tolerated with minimal adverse events.
Llufriu et al. [40]	41 patients Median age: 33 (range 14–57) 61% female Diagnoses: MS 56% (23), ADEM 17% (7), NMO 10% (4), CIS 5% (2), Marburg MS 5% (2), idiopathic ON 5% (2), idiopathic transverse myelitis 2% (1) Most had motor deficits: paraparesis (44%), quadriparesis, brainstem, or ON	• PLEX median of 6 sessions (range 5–15), every other day • Volume: 1.25–1.66 plasma volumes/ session • Replacement fluid: 5% albumin • Machine: Cobe Spectra (centrifugation) • Concomitant therapy: All had prior IV methylprednisolone (1 g/day × 3–5 days); 6 patients received IV steroids during PE; 2 received mitoxantrone; 7 received IVIg (200 mg/kg) post-PE sessions • Timing: PE started median 27 days from symptom onset (range 6–90)	• At discharge (median 12 days post-PE): 16 patients (39%) improved (15 EDSS, 1 VA) • At 6 months: 26 patients (63%) improved (23 EDSS, 3 VA) • EDSS improvement median: −2.5 (range − 1 to −7.5) • Response by timing: <15 days: 83%; 16–60 days: 67%; >60 days: 43% • Subgroup response rates at 6 months: MS 52%, ADEM 86%, NMO 75%, Marburg 50%, ON 75%, TM 100% • Adverse events: 24% hypotension, 5% bacteremia, 2% thrombosis, 2% rash	• Efficacy: PE is an effective rescue therapy in pediatric patients with steroid-refractory demyelinating diseases. • Predictors of response: Early PE initiation (<30 days post-relapse) and presence of gadolinium-enhancing MRI lesions significantly increased success rates. • Safety: Procedure is safe, with most complications being mild and manageable. • Clinical implications: Supports PLEX as a second-line option for pediatric MS and other demyelinating syndromes when steroids fail.

Study	N/ cohorts	Therapeutic Protocol	Results	Findings
Mesaros et al. [15]	107 MS patients with 127 severe relapses treated with PLEX. Phenotypes: 83.2% RRMS, 12.1% SPMS, 4.7% PPMS. Mean age: 39.2 years; Female-to-male ratio: 2.3:1.	• PLEX Protocol: 5–7 sessions over 14–21 days (median plasma volume: 1.0 per session). • Replacement fluids: Albumin and crystalloid solutions (e.g., saline). • Prior IV corticosteroids (99.3%).	• Clinical improvement: 73.8% marked improvement, 7.1% mild improvement, 19.0% no response. • EDSS improved significantly: Median reduced from 6.0 (nadir) to 4.0 (discharge). • Sustained improvement at 6 months ($p < 0.0001$). • Adverse events in 17.3% (e.g., hypotension, hypoalbuminemia).	• Predictors of positive outcomes: Younger age and lower EDSS at relapse nadir significantly associated with better response ($p < 0.05$). • Delay in PLEX initiation (median 32 days) did not significantly affect outcomes. • Safety: Adverse events were mild and manageable.
Weiner et al. [12]	116 patients experiencing severe, acute MS attacks. Randomized into active (PLEX) or sham groups. Mean Age: 37 years Predominantly female (70%).	• PLEX: 7 sessions over 14 days. • Plasma replaced with 5% albumin. • Sham Exchange: Blood separated and returned without plasma exchange. • Immunosuppression: ACTH or cyclophosphamide given to all patients.	• No statistically significant overall improvement between PLEX and sham ($p > 0.05$). • Subgroup analysis: Marginal improvement in relapsing-remitting MS with PLEX ($p = 0.06$). • Progressive MS showed no benefit. • Adverse Events: Mild: Hypotension, anemia. Severe: Thrombocytopenia, catheter-related infections.	• Efficacy: median time to recover was significantly shorter in the PLEX-treated patients; EDSS scores remained increased by 0.79 in the sham-treated group at 3 months. • Potential benefit in relapsing-remitting MS subgroup. • Safety: PLEX generally well-tolerated, but with risks of minor complications. • Conclusion: Findings suggest PLEX may have limited efficacy; further research is needed to identify responsive subgroups.

Abbreviations: ACTH, adrenocorticotropic hormone; ADEM, acute disseminated encephalomyelitis; AZA, azathioprine; BW, body weight; CIDP, chronic inflammatory demyelinating polyneuropathy; CIS, clinically isolated syndrome; CR, complete response; CVC, central venous catheter; CYCLO, cyclophosphamide; DSS, disability status scale; EDSS, expanded disability status score; FFP, fresh frozen plasma; GBS, Guillain-Barré syndrome; GCS, glucocorticoids; IM, intramuscular; IQR, interquartile range; IV, intravenous; MG, myasthenia gravis; MOGAD, myelin oligodendrocyte glycoprotein antibody disease; MP, methylprednisolone; MRI, magnetic resonance imaging; MS, multiple sclerosis; NMO, neuromyelitis optica; NR, no response; PNS, peripheral neuropathy syndrome; PPMS, primary progressive multiple sclerosis; PR, partial response; PV, plasma volume; RRMS, relapsing remitting multiple sclerosis; SPMS, secondary progressive multiple sclerosis; PLEX, therapeutic plasma exchange A. PLEX for Acute MS.

Table 1.
Clinical trials of PLEX in MS.

4.1 PLEX for progressive MS

While its use is well established in acute forms of MS, emerging evidence suggests that PLEX may also provide therapeutic benefit in progressive forms of MS, particularly in patients experiencing superimposed relapses or those with specific inflammatory profiles. In a double-blind, sham-controlled, randomized study of PLEX with or without low-dose immunosuppression (oral prednisone and cyclophosphamide), patients with chronic progressive MS demonstrated durable clinical improvement, with some patient showing sustained improvement in EDSS for up to 1 year [10]. Improvements in function were sustained in a 25-year follow-up study, some patients had not received any immunosuppressive drugs [13]. Notably, treatment benefits were more pronounced in patients with shorter disease duration and in those who had declined in their disability in the previous 2 years. A meta-analysis further supported the potential benefit of PLEX in progressive MS [27]. By analyzing data from six clinical trials, the study found that patients receiving PLEX had significantly reduced risk of neurological decline at 12 months compared to those who received standard of care or sham treatment.

A double-blind, sham-controlled, randomized study conducted by the Canadian Cooperative MS Group [26] evaluated the efficacy of PLEX in patients with progressive MS. The primary analysis compared the rates of treatment failure (worsening of EDSS score) among the groups. The study found no significant differences in treatment failure rates or other outcome measures among the groups. However, there was frequent and uncontrolled use of corticosteroids in patients who worsened clinically, thereby confounding the interpretation of the results. Patients who received corticosteroids due to clinical worsening of symptoms were *not* classified as "treatment failure." A total of 21/56 patients in the placebo group received corticosteroids, whereas only 8/56 in the treatment group did. When corticosteroids were controlled for in the analysis, the Canadian Study acknowledged that PLEX significantly ($p = 0.005$) delayed the time to treatment failure. A PLEX protocol to treat progressive MS is described in **Table 2**.

4.2 PLEX in the pediatric population

Pediatric MS is a less common form of MS, accounting for about 3–5% of all MS cases, and can be particularly severe as children may experience faster disability progression compared to adults with MS. People who develop MS early in life appear to be vulnerable to heightened inflammation and axonal loss [44]. At the same time, their younger age may provide protection through the brain's enhanced compensatory abilities [45, 46].

In the United States, fingolimod (Gilenya™) is currently the only Food and Drug Administration (FDA)-approved DMT for the treatment of relapsing MS in children and adolescents aged 10 years and older. While other DMTs like interferon-beta and glatiramer acetate are commonly used in adults with MS, their use in pediatric patients is considered "off-label" until further research and FDA approval are obtained. Teriflunomide is also approved for pediatric MS in some parts of the world, but not in the United States.

Although PLEX is less commonly applied in pediatric populations compared to adults, it holds significant promise, especially for children experiencing severe demyelinating relapses or recurrent relapses. In these cases, PLEX can serve as an alternative to frequent corticosteroid pulses, thus reducing the cumulative side effects associated with prolonged steroid use. One case report described a 7-year-old MS patient with high titers of antinuclear autoantibodies who demonstrated marked improvement following PLEX, highlighting its potential as a life-altering intervention

Disease state	Induction phase	Tapering/Maintenance phase
For an acute MS attack	One plasma volume* TPE at an intensity of 2–3 procedures per week for 2 weeks. Replacement fluid would be 5% albumin.**	Once weekly and then gradually tapered and is continued as dictated by the patient's response. PLEX is discontinued once improved and stabilized.
For progressive and secondary progressive MS	One plasma volume, once a week for 10 weeks. Replacement fluid would be 5% albumin.	Gradually taper as determined by the clinical response. May require mPLEX*** (Typically, once every 4 to 8 weeks).
Fulminant or malignant MS, tumefactive MS, Marburg variant	Up to 5 PLEX procedures for 1 week then 3 PLEX procedures for 1 week. Replacement fluid would be 5% albumin.	Once weekly then gradually tapered as dictated by the clinical response. Many patients will require ongoing mPLEX (typically once every 4 to 8 weeks).
Post PLEX Supplement Replacements	Cyanocobalamin 1000mcg IM post treatment. For 2 or more PLEX a week, administer weekly at the end of the week. For PLEX once a week, administer at every 5th procedure. Folic acid 1 mg daily while on PLEX.	
Anticoagulation	Citrate dextrose solution A 1:10. Add calcium gluconate 0.2 gm to each 250 ml of replacement fluid.	

**One plasma volume PLEX is approximately 3000 ml. For example, for a patient weighing 70 kg with a 40% hematocrit, 3 liters of plasma is processed per procedure.*
***Replacement fluid should include plasma in patients with conditions such as TTP, in those in the perioperative period, or those who have bleeding disorders or are at high risk of bleeding.*
****Maintenance PLEX.*
Abbreviations: IM, intramuscular; MS, multiple sclerosis; TPE, therapeutic plasma exchange.

Table 2.
PLEX Protocol Recommendations.

in select pediatric cases [47]. Additionally, Tenembaum and colleagues assessed the role of PLEX in pediatric patients with severe demyelinating CNS events unresponsive to corticosteroids [48]. Among the 41 children treated, 63% showed clinical improvement at 6 months, with 39% achieving marked recovery. The study further supports the use of PLEX as an effective and safe second-line therapy in pediatric populations with steroid-resistant relapses.

5. Maintenance PLEX

Patients with relapsing or progressive MS who respond to initial PLEX may need ongoing maintenance therapy, as demonstrated by the following examples of real patient histories.

A. Long-term treatment success with PLEX.

For patients with chronic autoimmune diseases like MS, ongoing therapy is typically required. Although PLEX will not cure chronic autoimmune conditions, patients can experience long-term disease control if appropriately managed on a PLEX maintenance program.

Patient #1 (Video 1 https://bit.ly/4ln2Qgx*):* A 26-year-old male was diagnosed with severe MS in 1996. Despite injectable interferon and intravenous methylprednisolone, he remained wheelchair-bound, unable to transfer or feed himself. Choking led to aspiration pneumonia and extended hospital stays. PLEX was initiated in Nov 1999, initially twice a week for 3 weeks, then tapering to once every 6 weeks. By 6 years, he was able to walk without assistance, could do tandem gait, and could hop on one leg. He has been solely on maintenance PLEX for the past 25 years.

B. Insurance approval as a determinant of access to PLEX.

Despite the emphasis on evidence-based medicine in physician training, insurance approval can often be a significant limitation as to how patients are treated. Even with convincing published data, insurance companies either deny PLEX or approve it only for an acute exacerbation when other treatments have failed. Maintenance PLEX therapy, which could potentially allow patients to discontinue long-term immunosuppressive drugs and avoid their side effect profiles, is usually not approved even if the patient initially responds well to PLEX. This often leads to patients having to take chronic steroid medication, which can cause complications such as Cushingoid features, osteoporosis, hypertension, and diabetes, as seen in patients with CIDP and MG. On the other hand, maintenance PLEX therapy (typically once a month) could potentially allow them to discontinue steroids and avoid such complications.

Patient #2 (Video 2 https://bit.ly/4ln2Qgx*):* In 1994, a 27-year-old Caucasian woman was significantly disabled due to worsening of her MS and was started on weekly PLEX with remarkable improvement. She returned to work and continued to improve while on maintenance PLEX until 1996 when it was discontinued due to insurance denial. This led to regression and 2 years in a wheelchair, despite ACTH, steroids, and cyclophosphamide. Multiple appeals led to reapproval of PLEX, and she was able to walk independently and return to work within 8 months. In 2003, PLEX was again denied, and she became wheelchair bound. With PLEX reapproved in 2004, she improved and was able to walk across a room independently. When her PLEX treatments were once again denied by her insurance company, she regressed and is now (as of 2021) quadriparetic. Maintenance PLEX was never approved; natalizumab was approved but did not improve her condition.

6. Predictors of favorable response to PLEX

Several predictors of favorable response have been identified, including:

6.1 Time to initiation

A shorter interval between relapse onset and PLEX initiation significantly improves outcomes. Most responders exhibit improvement within a median of 4 days or after the third PLEX procedure [2, 40, 49, 50].

6.2 Baseline disability

Patients with lower pre-treatment EDSS scores are more likely to achieve better recovery. Shorter disease duration prior to PLEX initiation correlates with better outcomes, reflecting the importance of early intervention [36]. In progressive MS the degree of decline in EDSS in relation to the time at which treatment was initiated was noted to be a significant predictor of improvement [51]. Seventy-five percent of patients who improved were treated within a year from the time of their decline on EDSS by one or more steps. The severity of disability just prior to PLEX did not seem to influence the outcome in this study. The mean improvement that occurred was proportionally the same in patients at different EDSS levels just prior to treatment.

6.3 MRI features

Radiographic features, particularly gadolinium-enhancing (Gd+) magnetic resonance imaging (MRI) lesions, strongly predict PLEX response. Patients with large (>2 cm) tumefactive or ring-enhancing lesions are more likely to benefit. Among these, nearly 52% exhibited ring-enhancing lesions on MRI, which were significantly associated with favorable outcomes [36, 50].

6.4 Additional clinical predictors

Preserved deep tendon reflexes and early symptomatic improvement during PLEX sessions are associated with better outcomes [30].

7. Procedure for PLEX administration

PLEX is a procedure in which the patient's blood is passed through an apheresis machine, where the separated patient plasma is removed and discarded with reinfusion of patient cellular blood components along with replacement fluid such as donor plasma or albumin into the patient. It is performed as described below, and practical considerations are presented in **Box 1**.

1. Avoid spinal tap or any invasive or surgical procedures at least 24 hours before and after the procedure because the use of anticoagulation and PLEX itself may transiently affect bleeding and clotting time, especially if the replacement fluid does not replace coagulation factors.

2. Administer routine medications after PLEX if possible since some of the drugs may be removed from circulation during the procedure.

3. For PLEX procedures planned for an extended period, the replacement fluid should be 5% albumin.

4. To mitigate citrate toxicity due to acid citrate dextrose, give IV calcium in the replacement fluid or oral calcium carbonate.

5. Videotape all your patients before and after PLEX to monitor progress and, if necessary, to share with the insurance company if there is a coverage denial in the future. Patients often forget how much they were suffering prior to starting PLEX, a so-called 'point-of-reference phenomenon' which is quite common following improved functioning or symptom mitigation.

6. Avoid placement of in-dwelling central lines and use peripheral access whenever possible (including temporary radial or brachial arteries). This technique is safe, quick, and easy to learn.

7. Educate your peers, nurses, and patients on the value of PLEX. Pharmaceutical companies spend a lot of money and resources to promote their products. They make sure that all healthcare providers (and patients) are targeted through advertising in medical journals, office visits, at conferences, peer-to-peer talks, and through social media. Comparatively, very little marketing is done for PLEX.

Box 1.
Practical Considerations for Incorporating PLEX in a Clinical Practice

7.1 Steps

- Patient lies comfortably in a bed or is seated in a chair.
- A BD angiocath 16-gauge catheter is inserted into a blood vessel such as an antecubital vein.
- The blood is pulled through this catheter into the PLEX machine.
- The blood is circulated through an apheresis instrument that separates the patient's plasma from the remaining cellular blood components.
- The patient's plasma is discarded, and a replacement fluid, such as albumin, is added to the blood cells.
- The patient's cellular blood components and replacement fluid are returned to the patient through a BD 18-gauge catheter inserted into a peripheral vein. PLEX takes about 2 to 3 hours, depending on the amount of patient plasma that needs to be removed.

8. PLEX versus immunoadsorption

In cases where steroids fail to be effective, alternative treatments like PLEX and immunoadsorption (IA) can be effective. Although effective, PLEX can lead to adverse events (AEs), such as hypotension, allergic reactions, anticoagulation-related issues like hypocalcemia, or bleeding due to removal of coagulation factors. In contrast, IA is a more precise method that targets antibody removal while leaving other plasma components intact, which may offer a better safety profile. This distinction has made IA an increasingly popular alternative for treating certain neurological conditions. Both techniques have demonstrated success in treating steroid-resistant MS relapses. However, direct comparisons of their outcomes, safety, and overall tolerability remain limited. The choice between PLEX and IA often depends on factors such as instrument type availability, the procedures involved, the treatment protocols, and the unique needs of each patient.

In a study by Dorst and colleagues, 284 patients with various autoimmune neurological diseases, including MS, received either PLEX or IA [52]. While both modalities demonstrated similar efficacy in improving clinical outcomes, IA was associated with a significantly higher rate of mild to moderate AEs, such as hypotension and allergic reactions. Severe AEs were rare in both groups, but the overall safety profile favored PLEX due to its lower incidence of complications. Consistent with these results, a retrospective study of 140 patients with MS or neuromyelitis optica (NMO) who underwent either PLEX or IA showed comparable efficacy between the two treatments in managing steroid-refractory relapses [53]. However, the study identified several predictors of better response, including younger age, female sex, central venous access, and earlier initiation of apheresis. These findings highlight the potential for individualized treatment decisions based on patient characteristics and logistical considerations. Indeed, a systematic review of 63 studies examining the use of PLEX and IA in acute demyelinating diseases also revealed both modalities demonstrate comparable efficacy, with response rates ranging from 42 to 90% for PLEX and 50 to 86% for IA [31]. Importantly, early initiation of apheresis correlated with better clinical outcomes, reinforcing the need for timely escalation in refractory cases.

9. Vascular access considerations for PLEX procedures

Vascular access is a critical component of PLEX, and the selection of an appropriate access method can significantly influence both procedural success and patient safety. PLEX requires adequate vascular access for removing blood from circulation (usually at the rate of 60–100 mL per minute) and typically with another venous access to return cells and replacement fluid to the circulation.

Peripheral vascular access (PVA) is often underutilized despite its numerous advantages, particularly in terms of safety and cost-effectiveness. Peripheral catheters, typically 17- to 19-gauge for adults, can achieve sufficient flow rates for PLEX, especially with centrifuge-based systems requiring flow rates of 50 to 120 mL/minute. While smaller-gauge catheters may limit flow in pediatric patients, PVA still offers a feasible option in many cases. Single-needle techniques can also be used when only one venous site is available, although they generally extend procedure time.

PVA presents several advantages, including immediate usability, low infection risk, cost-efficiency, and the ability for general nursing staff to place and remove the access. However, limitations include a greater need for patient cooperation, potential for bruising or superficial thrombophlebitis, risk of access loss mid-procedure, and suboptimal applicability in certain populations such as in pediatric or psychiatric patients or in those with poor vein integrity.

While PVA is preferred, many patients usually require an indwelling central line or embedded ports for vascular access to perform PLEX. This approach is a leading cause of serious complications related to PLEX [54]. One center uses strictly all central lines for vascular access and has experienced complications in 20% of their patients. These complications include infection, thrombosis, bleeding, and catheter kinking. At other centers, outflow vascular access is successfully accomplished by placing a 16-gauge angio-catheter in an antecubital vein. The placement of an arterial catheter takes just a few minutes and may be facilitated with use of an ultrasound machine for easier placement. However, in about one-third of the patients this approach fails. In these patients, a temporary 18-gauge arterial catheter is inserted in the radial (preferred) or brachial artery which usually allows a blood flow of 80 to 120 mL/minute (*Video 3* https://bit.ly/4ln2Qgx *without ultrasound assistance, Video 4* https://bit.ly/4ln2Qgx *with ultrasound assistance*) [55]. The catheter is removed at the conclusion of the PLEX procedure and pressure is applied at the site until it stops bleeding. Rarely, it may require an ice bag over the site to stop bleeding. A pressure bandage is applied, which can be removed by the patient typically 4 hours later. The return line is via an 18-gauge angio-catheter placed peripherally in a vein, not on the same arm as the outflow access. A tourniquet is placed above the venous access; a heating pad is placed over it; and the patient is asked to squeeze off and on, ensuring adequate blood flow.

One of the physician's assistants, who had never inserted an arterial catheter before, learned how to do this procedure within a week. She now routinely inserts them via ultrasound-guidance in patients. This process is applied at each PLEX procedure, takes less than 5 minutes, and one author (BOK) has thus far inserted over 20,000 temporary radial or brachial artery catheters without any major complications. In a few patients who required long-term maintenance PLEX, we have inserted a temporary catheter in the radial or brachial artery over 400 times, in each, without any complications.

Based on our experience and that of others, and in keeping with the American Society for Apheresis Choosing Wisely recommendations [56], we avoid use of central venous vascular access options whenever possible. Indwelling central line catheters are associated with serious complications, such as infection and thrombosis. In a handful of patients over the years, in whom PVA and arterial access was difficult, we have used an indwelling central line using Permcath™ chronic silicone oval catheter. It provides an average blood flow rates of 400 mL/min. Ports or fistula for vascular access can also be utilized in certain patients.

10. Safety of PLEX

Automated apheresis devices have been used in clinical care since the 1980s. Since then, therapeutic apheresis (TA), including PLEX, has been shown to be safe, with an overall AE rate below 3%. PLEX remains a viable option for critically ill patients and those with comorbidities for whom conventional therapies may be contraindicated. Clinical evidence supports the safety of PLEX for treating demyelinating and neuro-immunological conditions, including MS. Registries report large numbers of patients and procedures [57–59], and their regular reports show that apheresis procedures are generally quite safe, with a low total AE rate and severe AE rates of 0.1–0.15%. The procedure-related mortality rate is extremely low (<0.007%).

The risk profile of PLEX varies based on both modifiable and unmodifiable factors. Modifiable risks associated with PLEX include those related to the procedure itself, such as citrate toxicity, hypotension, and hypocalcemia, which can be managed with calcium supplementation and careful monitoring. Other modifiable risks include allergic reactions to replacement fluids and ensuring proper vascular access. All these AEs are transient and readily correctable. Unmodifiable factors include:

1. Age of patient. While PLEX is generally considered safe across age groups, the youngest and oldest patients may have a slightly higher risk of complications compared to adults, though these are often mild and manageable.

2. Disease severity. PLEX is well tolerated in patients who are critically ill with renal and heart failure and respirator dependent [60], in septic shock [61], and immunocompromised status [62].

3. Procedure frequency and total volume exchanged is important to focus on to avoid adverse events. Typically, 1.0 to 1.5 plasma volumes are exchanged per session. Less than one plasma volume may be ineffective, and exceeding 1.5 plasma volumes may increase risk without added benefit. Pediatric patients require special attention due to smaller blood volumes and associated slightly higher complication risk.

4. Baseline lab values. PLEX is safe in renal failure, patients with cancer [63] and safe and effective bridging therapy for patients with acute liver failure and acute-on-chronic liver failure [64].

11. Underutilization of PLEX in the United States

Despite clinical data supporting the use of PLEX for MS, in the United States, PLEX is generally used as a last resort for neurological conditions when other treatments have failed or proven to be ineffective. This decision is driven largely by insurance policy makers and to a lesser extent by healthcare providers who may not have sufficient experience in the use of PLEX or because of difficult access to this procedure. Based on our over 40 years of experience with 70,000 PLEX procedures for treating patients with severe neurological disorders, we have come to view it as a viable and effective first line of defense rather than a "last resort" or "rescue therapy". The safety of the procedure in the long term supports its use in lifelong diseases like MS. In addition, we have clinically observed nine patients who have been continuously treated with PLEX for the past 30 years (frequency once every 6 to 8 weeks). These patients were severely disabled for an extended period, despite trying all conventional treatments; but because of PLEX, they became, and remain, fully ambulatory.

When used early in the course of disease or during an acute exacerbation, PLEX can bring about rapid improvement. However, instead of continuing with the therapy, clinicians often choose to abruptly stop PLEX after rendering five to seven treatments in 1 or 2 weeks. This, we believe, is a mistake. Quite often it takes frequent treatments (once or twice weekly for 5 weeks for an acute event, and once a week for 10 weeks for a progressive disease) to notice improvement. In either situation, if there is a noticeable improvement, PLEX should be continued over a longer period while gradually decreasing its frequency. Some patients may need ongoing maintenance PLEX therapy for a considerable length of time. Insurance companies quite often deny maintenance therapy, even when the patient had improved after a short course of PLEX.

12. Comparison of PLEX and approved high-efficacy therapies in MS

When evaluating the safety in treating RRMS, it is appropriate to consider the rates and severity of AEs associated with PLEX in the context of other approved and/or widely used MS drug therapies. Some of the most used immunotherapies for MS, include B cell-depleting drugs such as ocrelizumab, ublituximab, and ofatumumab, while other classes of drugs include natalizumab and cladribine [65]. Ocrelizumab was the first drug in that B cell-depleting class, approved in 2017, while natalizumab, cladribine, ofatumumab, and ublituximab were approved in 2004, 2019, 2020, and 2022 respectively. Since the first drug approvals, there have been robust reporting on AEs and complications arising from their use (**Table 3**) [66].

Some of these drugs can cause significant lymphopenia and hypogammaglobulinemia putting the patients at the risk for serious infections [67–69]. There are known risks of reactivation of latent or occult infections, and published recommendations advise careful screening and monitoring for potentially serious disease mediators like herpes virus, John Cunningham virus (JC virus), human papilloma virus, hepatitis B (HBV), hepatitis C (HBC), tuberculosis, and cytomegalovirus (CMV) [70]. Rare but serious side effect of immunotherapy includes the risk of progressive multifocal leukoencephalopathy (PML), which can be fatal, and there is no known therapy for this [71–73]. Additionally, acute liver injury and reactivation of HBV are listed risks for several common immunosuppressive therapies [74] As such, hepatic screening tests and regular monitoring during therapy is recommended. Additionally, there is insufficient guidance based on long-term data to inform how long a patient may safely receive these drugs. In contrast, PLEX has no such risk factors and can be safely used on a long-term basis.

DOI: http://dx.doi.org/10.5772/intechopen.1010410

Therapy	Long term safety	Significant risks for procedure or drug	Black box warning	Risk of teratogenicity
PLEX	Safe	• Transient: hypocalcemia • Hypotension • Transfusion reactions • Fluid and electrolyte imbalance • Hypofibrinogenemia • Thrombocytopenia	No	No
IVIG	Safe	• Acute kidney injury • Venous thrombosis • Aseptic meningitis • Hemolytic anemia • TRALI • Transfusion reaction	No	No
Cladribine	Not known	• Upper respiratory tract infections • Malignancies • Teratogenicity • Serious infections including PML • Anemia • Cardiac failure • Serious liver injury	Malignancy, Teratogenicity	Yes
Natalizumab	Risk of PML	• Transfusion reaction • Serious infections including PML • Serious liver injury • Lower respiratory tract infections	PML	Yes
Ocrelizumab	Not known	• Transfusion reaction • Serious infections including PML • Malignancies • Upper and lower respiratory tract infections	No	Yes
Ofatumumab	Not known	• Injection reaction • Upper respiratory infections • Reactivation: PML, HBV • Serious opportunistic infections • Fetal risks	No	Yes
Ublituximab	Not known	• Infusion reaction • Serious infections, including HBV and PML • Upper respiratory tract infections • Hypogammaglobulinemia • Fetal risks	No	Yes

Abbreviations: HBV, hepatitis B virus; MS, multiple sclerosis; PML, progressive multifocal leukoencephalopathy; TRALI, transfusion-related acute lung injury.

Table 3.
Drug Manufacturer Published Risks. Published warnings for FDA-approved drugs for MS include increased risk of hematologic toxicity, hepatotoxicity, and malignancy. Data obtained from manufacturers' websites, accessed 01/09/2025.

PLEX is less expensive than currently used biologics. The charge for one PLEX procedure in 2021 at our institution was approximately $5000.00. In comparison, one single ocrelizumab infusion was $106,720.00 and one natalizumab infusion was $24,170.00.

13. Conclusion

PLEX is a safe and effective therapy both for acute and chronic progressive MS patients unresponsive to conventional therapies. We have yet to identify evidence-based contraindications in patients for whom PLEX is indicated. Patients in septic shock; hepatic, renal or heart failure; acute stroke; respiratory crisis; and patients of practically any age have tolerated and responded well to PLEX [75]. It is a fast-acting immunomodulator, does not cause immunosuppression, and has a highly favorable long-term safety record in both an outpatient and inpatient settings. In patients with significant comorbidities or who are acutely ill, or in those who have a fulminant autoimmune attack, PLEX would be our first choice over drugs associated with immunosuppression. It is important to use a disease state appropriate PLEX protocol and, in particular, not undertreat conditions that are responding to PLEX therapy. Most complications associated with PLEX are related to indwelling central venous catheter (CVC). While alternative vascular access options such as fully implanted apheresis-compatible ports are available, we cannot overemphasize the importance of avoiding an indwelling central line access whenever possible. PLEX is less expensive than currently used biopharmaceutical, and advantages in clinical impacts with PLEX may be due to its unique mechanisms of action. Along with insurance denials, a lack of appreciation of how PLEX can benefit MS in a main reason for its underutilization. Finally, if you are a neurologist with an interest in treating auto-immune neurological disorders, invest in having your own PLEX program or closely partner with a team which operates an existing one.

Acknowledgements

Grant support for publication fees was provided by Terumo Blood and Cell Technologies.

Disclosures

BOK: Bristol-Meyer Squibb, Sanofi, Genentech, Biogen, Alexion, TG Therapeutics, EMD Serono. UCB. Argenix, Terumo BCT.

JSR: consultant for Sanofi, Genzyme; American Society for Apheresis Board of Directors Member.

Additional materials

Video materials referenced in this chapter are available online at: https://bit.ly/4ln2Qgx

Author details

Bhupendra O. Khatri[1*] and Jay S. Raval[2]

1 The Regional Multiple Sclerosis Center, Center for Neurological Disorders, S. C., St. Francis Hospital, Milwaukee, WI, USA

2 University of Vermont, Medical Center, Robert Larner College of Medicine, Department of Pathology and Medicine, Burlington, VT, USA

*Address all correspondence to: milwaukee4145@gmail.com

References

[1] The North American study of plasmapheresis in the Guillain-Barre syndrome. The Guillain-Barre' syndrome study group. Journal of Clinical Apheresis. 1985;**2**(4):315-320. DOI: 10.1002/jca.2920020416

[2] Bonnan M, Cabre P. Plasma exchange in severe attacks of neuromyelitis optica. Multiple Sclerosis International. 2012; **2012**:787630. DOI: 10.1155/2012/787630

[3] Dau PC. Plasmapheresis therapy in myasthenia gravis. Muscle & Nerve. 1980;**3**(6):468-482. DOI: 10.1002/mus.880030603

[4] Guillevin L. Plasma exchanges. A still effective treatment. Presse Médicale. 2019;**48**(11 Pt. 2):317-318. DOI: 10.1016/j.lpm.2019.11.007

[5] Hahn AF et al. Plasma-exchange therapy in chronic inflammatory demyelinating polyneuropathy. A double-blind, sham-controlled, cross-over study. Brain. 1996;**119**(Pt. 4): 1055-1066. DOI: 10.1093/brain/119.4.1055

[6] Hiew FL et al. Consensus recommendation on the use of therapeutic plasma exchange for adult neurological diseases in Southeast Asia from the Southeast Asia therapeutic plasma exchange consortium. Journal of Central Nervous System Disease. 2021; **13**:11795735211057314. DOI: 10.1177/11795735211057314

[7] Jacob S, Mazibrada G, Irani SR, Jacob A, Yudina A. The role of plasma exchange in the treatment of refractory autoimmune neurological diseases: A narrative review. Journal of Neuroimmune Pharmacology. 2021; **16**(4):806-817. DOI: 10.1007/s11481-021-10004-9

[8] Kambara C, Matsuo H, Fukudome T, Goto H, Shibuya N. Miller fisher syndrome and plasmapheresis. Therapeutic Apheresis. 2002;**6**(6): 450-453. DOI: 10.1046/j.1526-0968.2002.00466.x

[9] Khatri BO, Kramer J, Dukic M, Palencia M, Verre W. Maintenance plasma exchange therapy for steroid-refractory neuromyelitis optica. Journal of Clinical Apheresis. 2012;**27**(4): 183-192. DOI: 10.1002/jca.21215

[10] Khatri BO, McQuillen MP, Harrington GJ, Schmoll D, Hoffmann RG. Chronic progressive multiple sclerosis: Double-blind controlled study of plasmapheresis in patients taking immunosuppressive drugs. Neurology. 1985;**35**(3):312-319. DOI: 10.1212/wnl.35.3.312

[11] Osman C, Jennings R, El-Ghariani K, Pinto A. Plasma exchange in neurological disease. Practical Neurology. 2020;**20**(2): 92-99. DOI: 10.1136/practneurol-2019-002336

[12] Weiner HL et al. Double-blind study of true vs. sham plasma exchange in patients treated with immunosuppression for acute attacks of multiple sclerosis. Neurology. 1989; **39**(9):1143-1149. DOI: 10.1212/wnl.39.9.1143

[13] Khatri BO, Tarima S, McQuillen MP, Kramer J, Dukic M, Bellanger C. Plasma exchange in secondary progressive multiple sclerosis: Twenty-five year follow-up study. Journal of Multiple Sclerosis. 2014;**1**(1). DOI: 10.4172/jmso.1000102

[14] Simpson A, Mowry EM, Newsome SD. Early aggressive

treatment approaches for multiple sclerosis. Current Treatment Options in Neurology. 2021;**23**(7):19. DOI: 10.1007/s11940-021-00677-1

[15] Mesaros S et al. Beneficial therapeutic plasma exchange response in the treatment of severe relapses in patients with multiple sclerosis. Acta Neurologica Belgica. 2024;**124**(6): 1885-1890. DOI: 10.1007/s13760-024-02606-w

[16] Comi G et al. Role of B cells in multiple sclerosis and related disorders. Annals of Neurology. 2021;**89**(1):13-23. DOI: 10.1002/ana.25927

[17] Stone MJ, Bogen SA. Role of plasmapheresis in Waldenstrom's macroglobulinemia. Clinical Lymphoma, Myeloma & Leukemia. 2013;**13**(2): 238-240. DOI: 10.1016/j.clml.2013.02.013

[18] Rock GA et al. Comparison of plasma exchange with plasma infusion in the treatment of thrombotic thrombocytopenic purpura. Canadian apheresis study group. The New England Journal of Medicine. 1991;**325**(6): 393-397. DOI: 10.1056/NEJM199108083250604

[19] Chevret S, Hughes RA, Annane D. Plasma exchange for Guillain-Barre syndrome. Cochrane Database of Systematic Reviews. 2017;**2**(2): CD001798. DOI: 10.1002/14651858.CD001798.pub3

[20] Weinshenker BG et al. A randomized trial of plasma exchange in acute central nervous system inflammatory demyelinating disease. Annals of Neurology. 1999;**46**(6):878-886. DOI: 10.1002/1531-8249(199912)46:6<878::aid-ana10>3.0.co;2-q

[21] Reeves HM, Winters JL. The mechanisms of action of plasma exchange. British Journal of Haematology. 2014;**164**(3):342-351. DOI: 10.1111/bjh.12629

[22] Tindall RS, Walker JE, Ehle AL, Near L, Rollins J, Becker D. Plasmapheresis in multiple sclerosis: Prospective trial of pheresis and immunosuppression versus immunosuppression alone. Neurology. 1982;**32**(7):739-743. DOI: 10.1212/wnl.32.7.739

[23] Hauser SL et al. Intensive immunosuppression in progressive multiple sclerosis. A randomized, three-arm study of high-dose intravenous cyclophosphamide, plasma exchange, and ACTH. The New England Journal of Medicine. 1983;**308**(4):173-180. DOI: 10.1056/NEJM198301273080401

[24] Gordon PA et al. A double-blind controlled pilot study of plasma exchange versus sham apheresis in chronic progressive multiple sclerosis. The Canadian Journal of Neurological Sciences. 1985;**12**(1):39-44. DOI: 10.1017/s0317167100046564

[25] Khatri BO, Koethe SM, McQuillen MP. Plasmapheresis with immunosuppressive drug therapy in progressive multiple sclerosis. A pilot study. Archives of Neurology. 1984; **41**(7):734-738. DOI: 10.1001/archneur.1984.04050180056018

[26] The Canadian cooperative trial of cyclophosphamide and plasma exchange in progressive multiple sclerosis. The Canadian cooperative multiple sclerosis study group. Lancet. 1991;**337**(8739): 441-446 [Online]. Available from: https://www.ncbi.nlm.nih.gov/pubmed/1671468

[27] Vamvakas EC, Pineda AA, Weinshenker BG. Meta-analysis of clinical studies of the efficacy of plasma

exchange in the treatment of chronic progressive multiple sclerosis. Journal of Clinical Apheresis. 1995;**10**(4):163-170. DOI: 10.1002/jca.2920100402

[28] Linker RA et al. Plasma exchange therapy for steroid-refractory superimposed relapses in secondary progressive multiple sclerosis. Journal of Neurology. 2007;**254**(9):1288-1289. DOI: 10.1007/s00415-006-0497-0

[29] Grapsa E, Triantafyllou N, Rombos A, Lagouranis A, Dimopoulos MA. Therapeutic plasma exchange combined with immunomodulating agents in secondary progressive multiple sclerosis patients. Therapeutic Apheresis and Dialysis. 2008;**12**(2):105-108. DOI: 10.1111/j.1744-9987.2008.00554.x

[30] Magana SM et al. Beneficial plasma exchange response in central nervous system inflammatory demyelination. Archives of Neurology. 2011;**68**(7):870-878. DOI: 10.1001/archneurol.2011.34

[31] Rolfes L et al. Therapeutic apheresis in acute relapsing multiple sclerosis: Current evidence and unmet needs-a systematic review. Journal of Clinical Medicine. 2019;**8**(10). DOI: 10.3390/jcm8101623

[32] Ehler J et al. Treatment of the first acute relapse following therapeutic plasma exchange in formerly glucocorticosteroid-unresponsive multiple sclerosis patients-A Multicenter study to evaluate glucocorticosteroid responsiveness. International Journal of Molecular Sciences. 2017;**18**(8). DOI: 10.3390/ijms18081749

[33] Lehmann HC, Hartung HP, Hetzel GR, Stuve O, Kieseier BC. Plasma exchange in neuroimmunological disorders: Part 1: Rationale and treatment of inflammatory central nervous system disorders. Archives of Neurology. 2006;**63**(7):930-935. DOI: 10.1001/archneur.63.7.930

[34] Correia I et al. Plasma exchange in severe acute relapses of multiple sclerosis - results from a Portuguese cohort. Multiple Sclerosis and Related Disorders. 2018;**19**:148-152. DOI: 10.1016/j.msard.2017.12.001

[35] Keegan M, Pineda AA, McClelland RL, Darby CH, Rodriguez M, Weinshenker BG. Plasma exchange for severe attacks of CNS demyelination: Predictors of response. Neurology. 2002;**58**(1):143-146. DOI: 10.1212/wnl.58.1.143

[36] Ehler J et al. Response to therapeutic plasma exchange as a rescue treatment in clinically isolated syndromes and acute worsening of multiple sclerosis: A retrospective analysis of 90 patients. PLoS One. 2015;**10**(8):e0134583. DOI: 10.1371/journal.pone.0134583

[37] Korkmaz G et al. Effectiveness and safety of therapeutic plasma exchange in neurological diseases: An 11-year report from a tertiary care center. Therapeutic Apheresis and Dialysis. 2025;**29**(2):312-320. DOI: 10.1111/1744-9987.14223

[38] Bunganic R et al. Therapeutic plasma exchange in multiple sclerosis patients with an aggressive relapse: An observational analysis in a high-volume center. Scientific Reports. 2022;**12**(1):18374. DOI: 10.1038/s41598-022-23356-w

[39] Blechinger S et al. Therapeutic plasma exchange in steroid-refractory multiple sclerosis relapses. A retrospective two-center study. Therapeutic Advances in Neurological Disorders. 2021;**14**:1756286420975642. DOI: 10.1177/1756286420975642

[40] Llufriu S et al. Plasma exchange for acute attacks of CNS demyelination: Predictors of improvement at 6 months. Neurology. 2009;**73**(12):949-953. DOI: 10.1212/WNL.0b013e3181b879be

[41] Marques VD et al. Brazilian consensus for the treatment of multiple sclerosis: Brazilian academy of neurology and Brazilian committee on treatment and research in multiple sclerosis. Arquivos de Neuro-Psiquiatria. 2018; **76**(8):539-554. DOI: 10.1590/0004-282X20180078

[42] Cortese I, Chaudhry V, So YT, Cantor F, Cornblath DR, Rae-Grant A. Evidence-based guideline update: Plasmapheresis in neurologic disorders: Report of the therapeutics and technology assessment Subcommittee of the American Academy of Neurology. Neurology. 2011;**76**(3):294-300. DOI: 10.1212/WNL.0b013e318207b1f6

[43] Sellebjerg F et al. EFNS guideline on treatment of multiple sclerosis relapses: Report of an EFNS task force on treatment of multiple sclerosis relapses. European Journal of Neurology. 2005; **12**(12):939-946. DOI: 10.1111/j.1468-1331.2005.01352.x

[44] Pfeifenbring S et al. Extensive acute axonal damage in pediatric multiple sclerosis lesions. Annals of Neurology. 2015;**77**(4):655-667. DOI: 10.1002/ana.24364

[45] Rocca MA, Absinta M, Ghezzi A, Moiola L, Comi G, Filippi M. Is a preserved functional reserve a mechanism limiting clinical impairment in pediatric MS patients? Human Brain Mapping. 2009;**30**(9):2844-2851. DOI: 10.1002/hbm.20712

[46] Tortorella P et al. MRI quantification of gray and white matter damage in patients with early-onset multiple sclerosis. Journal of Neurology. 2006; **253**(7):903-907. DOI: 10.1007/s00415-006-0129-8

[47] Takahashi I, Sawaishi Y, Takeda O, Enoki M, Takada G. Childhood multiple sclerosis treated with plasmapheresis. Pediatric Neurology. 1997;**17**(1):83-87. DOI: 10.1016/s0887-8994(97)80673-x

[48] Tenembaum SN. Therapy of multiple sclerosis in children and adolescents. Clinical Neurology and Neurosurgery. 2010;**112**(7):633-640. DOI: 10.1016/j.clineuro.2010.04.015

[49] Huang X, Wu J, Xiao Y, Zhang Y. Timing of plasma exchange for neuromyelitis optica spectrum disorders: A meta-analysis. Multiple Sclerosis and Related Disorders. 2021;**48**:102709. DOI: 10.1016/j.msard.2020.102709

[50] Schilling S et al. Plasma exchange therapy for steroid-unresponsive multiple sclerosis relapses: Clinical experience with 16 patients. Nervenarzt. 2006;**77**(4):430-438. DOI: 10.1007/s00115-005-2019-1. Plasmaaustausch bei steroidresistenten Multiple-Sklerose-Schuben: Klinische Erfahrungen an 16 Patienten

[51] Khatri BO, McQuillen MP, Hoffmann RG, Harrington GJ, Schmoll D. Plasma exchange in chronic progressive multiple sclerosis: A long-term study. Neurology. 1991;**41**(3):409-414. DOI: 10.1212/wnl.41.3.409

[52] Dorst J, Fillies F, Dreyhaupt J, Senel M, Tumani H. Safety and tolerability of plasma exchange and immunoadsorption in neuroinflammatory diseases. Journal of Clinical Medicine. 2020;**9**(9). DOI: 10.3390/jcm9092874

[53] Lipphardt M et al. Immunoadsorption or plasma exchange

in steroid-refractory multiple sclerosis and neuromyelitis optica. Journal of Clinical Apheresis. 2019;**34**(4):381-391. DOI: 10.1002/jca.21686

[54] Rizvi MA et al. Complications of plasma exchange in 71 consecutive patients treated for clinically suspected thrombotic thrombocytopenic purpura-hemolytic-uremic syndrome. Transfusion. 2000;**40**(8):896-901. DOI: 10.1046/j.1537-2995.2000.40080896.x

[55] Khatri BO. Vascular access via temporary radial artery catheterization for therapeutic plasma exchange. Journal of Clinical Apheresis. 2003;**18**(3):134. DOI: 10.1002/jca.10060

[56] Connelly-Smith L et al. Choosing wisely for apheresis. Journal of Clinical Apheresis. 2018;**33**(5):576-579. DOI: 10.1002/jca.21643

[57] Wong ECC, Webb J, Pagano MB. The American Society for Apheresis (ASFA) disease registry: Past, present and future. Transfusion and Apheresis Science. 2017;**56**(6):779-782. DOI: 10.1016/j.transci.2017.11.027

[58] De Silvestro G et al. The Italian registry of therapeutic apheresis in SISTRA: Year of activity 2023. Transfusion and Apheresis Science. 2025;**64**(1):104037. DOI: 10.1016/j.transci.2024.104037

[59] Vrielink H et al. The world apheresis association registry, 2023 update. Transfusion and Apheresis Science. 2023;**62**(6):103831. DOI: 10.1016/j.transci.2023.103831

[60] Nusshag C et al. Plasma exchange in patients with severe coronavirus disease 2019: A single-Center experience. Critical Care Explorations. 2021;**3**(8): e0517. DOI: 10.1097/CCE.0000000000000517

[61] Knaup H et al. Early therapeutic plasma exchange in septic shock: A prospective open-label nonrandomized pilot study focusing on safety, hemodynamics, vascular barrier function, and biologic markers. Critical Care. 2018;**22**(1):285. DOI: 10.1186/s13054-018-2220-9

[62] Salim YS et al. Plasmaferesebehandling af perifer HIV-neuropati [Plasmapheresis in the treatment of peripheral HIV neuropathy]. Ugeskrift for Laeger. 1989; **151**(27):1754-1756 [Online]. Available from: https://www.ncbi.nlm.nih.gov/pubmed/2551089

[63] Hu Y, Yang H, Fu S, Wu J. Therapeutic plasma exchange: For cancer patients. Cancer Management and Research. 2022;**14**:411-425. DOI: 10.2147/CMAR.S340472

[64] Ramakrishnan S, Hans R, Duseja A, Sharma RR. Therapeutic plasma exchange is a safe and effective bridge therapy in patients with alcohol-associated ACLF not having immediate prospects for liver transplantation-a case-control, pilot study. Journal of Clinical Apheresis. 2022;**37**(6):553-562. DOI: 10.1002/jca.22010

[65] Chen C et al. Comparative efficacy and safety of disease-modifying therapies in patients with relapsing multiple sclerosis: A systematic review and network meta-analysis. Journal of the American Pharmaceutical Association. 2003, 2023;**63**(1):8-22 e23. DOI: 10.1016/j.japh.2022.07.009

[66] Sladowska K, Kawalec P, Holko P, Osiecka O. Comparative safety of high-efficacy disease-modifying therapies in relapsing-remitting multiple sclerosis: A systematic review and network meta-

analysis. Neurological Sciences. 2022; **43**(9):5479-5500. DOI: 10.1007/s10072-022-06197-3

[67] Alvarez E, Longbrake EE, Rammohan KW, Stankiewicz J, Hersh CM. Secondary hypogammaglobulinemia in patients with multiple sclerosis on anti-CD20 therapy: Pathogenesis, risk of infection, and disease management. Multiple Sclerosis and Related Disorders. 2023;**79**: 105009. DOI: 10.1016/j.msard.2023.105009

[68] Elgenidy A et al. Hypogammaglobulinemia and infections in patients with multiple sclerosis treated with anti-CD20 treatments: A systematic review and meta-analysis of 19,139 multiple sclerosis patients. Frontiers in Neurology. 2024;**15**:1380654. DOI: 10.3389/fneur.2024.1380654

[69] Fischer S, Proschmann U, Akgun K, Ziemssen T. Lymphocyte counts and multiple sclerosis therapeutics: Between mechanisms of action and treatment-limiting side effects. Cells. 2021;**10**(11). DOI: 10.3390/cells10113177

[70] Epstein DJ, Dunn J, Deresinski S. Infectious complications of multiple sclerosis therapies: Implications for screening, prophylaxis, and management. Open Forum Infectious Diseases. 2018;**5**(8):ofy174. DOI: 10.1093/ofid/ofy174

[71] Bloomgren G et al. Risk of natalizumab-associated progressive multifocal leukoencephalopathy. The New England Journal of Medicine. 2012; **366**(20):1870-1880. DOI: 10.1056/NEJMoa1107829

[72] Sharma K et al. Progressive multifocal leukoencephalopathy in anti-CD20 and other monoclonal antibody (mAb) therapies used in multiple sclerosis: A review. Journal of the Neurological Sciences. 2022;**443**:120459. DOI: 10.1016/j.jns.2022.120459

[73] Yousry TA et al. Evaluation of patients treated with natalizumab for progressive multifocal leukoencephalopathy. The New England Journal of Medicine. 2006;**354**(9): 924-933. DOI: 10.1056/NEJMoa054693

[74] Karvellas CJ et al. HBV-associated acute liver failure after immunosuppression and risk of death. Clinical Gastroenterology and Hepatology. 2017;**15**(1):113-122. DOI: 10.1016/j.cgh.2016.06.008

[75] Akcay N, Barlas UK, Bektas G, Kihtir HS, Sevketoglu E. Therapeutic plasma exchange in pediatric patients with acute demyelinating syndromes of the central nervous system: A single-center experience. Transfusion and Apheresis Science. 2022;**61**(4):103421. DOI: 10.1016/j.transci.2022.103421

Chapter 7

Cytoflavin in the Complex Therapy of Multiple Sclerosis

Sergey Mikhailovich Karpov and Irina Andreevna Vyshlova

Abstract

The article discusses the use of cytoflavin in the complex therapy of multiple sclerosis, as well as the use of evoked visual potentials for the diagnosis of this disease. The authors analyse the efficacy and safety of cytoflavin in the treatment of multiple sclerosis and discuss the possibilities of the method of evoked visual potentials in the detection and monitoring of patients with this disease. The results of the study may be useful for clinicians and researchers involved in the treatment and diagnosis of multiple sclerosis. They allow us to better understand the mechanisms of disease development and develop more effective methods of its treatment and prevention. The article is of interest to specialists in neurology, neurophysiology and other related fields, as well as to patients suffering from multiple sclerosis and their relatives.

Keywords: multiple sclerosis, diagnostic, treatment, visual evoked potentials, checkerboard pattern

1. Introduction

It has to be recognised that the number of patients with multiple sclerosis (MS) is now increasing annually. This problem covers practically all inhabitants of the world. There are difficulties in early diagnosis of MS. The use of visual evoked potentials (VEPs) for different colour spectra allows early detection of colour impulse disturbances in the visual analyser structures [1]. This technique is non-invasive, although it requires good training of health care workers to perform this test. In this regard, the use of evoked visual potentials in the early diagnosis of MS allows for early therapeutic measures, which makes it possible to avoid gross neurological defects in patients with MS.

2. Material and methods

The results of therapy of 41 patients diagnosed with MS, relapsing-remitting course, and exacerbation stage were analysed.

Inclusion criteria: established diagnosis of MS according to the revised McDonald criteria, relapsing-remitting type of course, age from 18 to 50 years, exacerbation stage lasting not more than 3 weeks, written informed consent [2].

IntechOpen

Exclusion criteria: taking antioxidants and neuroprotectants less than 2 weeks before the examination, refusal to sign informed consent.

The patients were randomised into two groups. The first group included 22 patients who received standard baseline therapy (methylprednisolone 1000 mg intravenous drip on 200 ml of physiological solution for 3-5 days), the second group consisted of 19 patients who in addition to baseline therapy received cytoflavin (LLC 'NTFF "POLISAN"', Russia) two tablets two times a day for a month.

All patients in dynamics (before the beginning of therapy, after 10 days and after treatment) were tested by clinical and laboratory examinations, assessment of neurological status using the functional systems scale (FSS) and expanded disability rating scale (EDSS), taking into account the results of neuroimaging (brain MRI) were performed [3].

Statistical processing of the material was performed by the method of variation statistics using the Microsoft Excel 2007 programme. Quantitative indices were evaluated for conformity to normal distribution using the Kolmogorov-Smirnov test, the difference between two groups – by Student's t-test, Mann-Whitney U-test. The results were statistically significant at $p < 0.05$.

2.1 Visual evoked potentials in the diagnosis of multiple sclerosis

The following clinical forms of the disease were identified from the total number of patients: RMS (relapsing multiple sclerosis)– 45 (56.9%) patients, SPMS (secondary progressive multiple sclerosis)– 15 (18.9%) patients, PPMS (primary progressive multiple sclerosis)– 19 (24.2%) patients.

Patients with RMS were predominant in the study group. In the group of patients with RMS, patients with a mild degree of disability prevailed. In the group of patients with SPMS, the number of patients with a moderate degree of disability increased 3-fold, and with a severe degree – 5.5-fold. In all groups of neurological symptoms, coordination disorders and central limb paresis were more common. In more than 90% of mild MS patients, only reflex disorders were observed. It is known that visual disturbances at one or another stage of the disease are detected in the overwhelming number of MS patients, and autopsy reveals optic nerve damage in 94-95% of cases. In this regard, the use of VEP determined a number of patterns in groups with different clinical forms of MS. An external stimulus with a different light spectrum was used. A black-and-white reversed checkerboard pattern is presented in **Figure 1**.

The results of the neurophysiological examination of MS patients for the black-and-white chess pattern are presented in **Table 1**.

Neurophysiological examination for black-and-white chess pattern allowed to reveal that the most significant reliable ($p < 0.01$) deviations in the parameters of VEP relative to the control group were observed in patients with SPMS and PPMS-clinical form. Thus, the latent period (LP) of the N75 wave in these forms was 85.3 ms, the index in RMSalso significantly ($p < 0.01$) differed from the parameters of the control group and was 81.81 ms (control group – 72.10.2 ms). The LP index of the most stable P100 wave was also sharply increased and differed significantly ($p < 0.001$) from that of the control group, being 127.09 ms at RMS, 128.3 ms at SPMS, and 124.5 ms at PPMS. (control group – 106.1 ms). LP far-field index (N 145) was also markedly ($p < 0.01$) increased. We noted that only 9 (15%) patients in the total sample (all cases in the group with RMS) had LP of the P100 waveform on the black-and-white pattern within the control group without significantly exceeding the control values. The results of descriptive statistics are presented in **Table 2**.

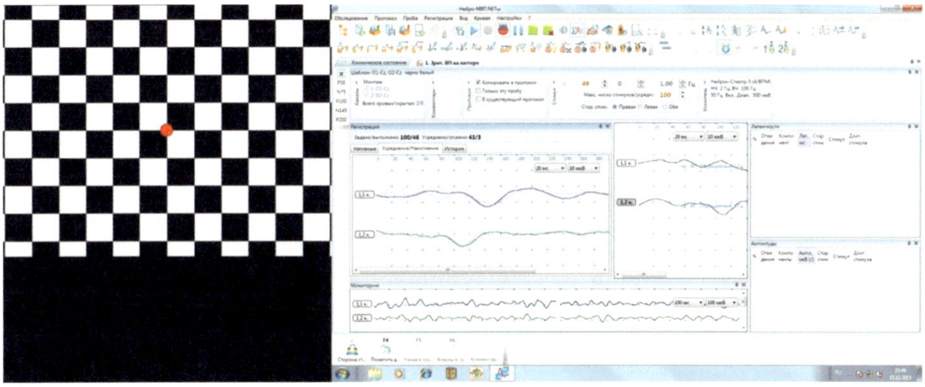

Figure 1.
Black-and-white reverse chess pattern.

VEP indices	RMS n = 31	SPMS n = 13	PPMS n = 16	Control group n = 31
Latent period (ms) N75 P100 N145 Amplitude (μV)	81,81 ± 0,79 [80,19-83,42]* 127,09 ± 0,85 [125,37-128,82]* 157,16 ± 1,03 [155,05-159,27]* 3,77 ± 0,4 [3,54-4,00]*	85,31 ± 0,80 [83,56-87,06]* 128,31 ± 1,06 [126,00-130,61]* 159,23 ± 1,16 [156,70-161,76]* 3,50 ± 0,7 [3,35-3,64]*	85,37 ± 0,67 [83,94-86,80]* 124,50 ± 1,50 [105,44-143,56]* 153,00 ± 1,00 [140,29-165,70]* 3,30 ± 0,15 [2,64-3,95]*	72,1 ± 0,2 106,1 ± 1,89 148,3 ± 1,41 8,5 ± 0,12
Spearman's correlation P100 wave	c SPMS -0,029 c PPMS +0,193 Contr. group −0,074	c PPMS +0,141 c RMS – 0,029 Contr. group +0,423	c RMS + 0,193 c SPMS +0,141 Contr. group +0,295	c RMS -0,074 c SPMS+0,423 c PPMS +0,295

95% confidence interval for the mean value.

Table 1.
Quantitative indices of VEP in patients with different clinical forms of MS per black/white chess pattern (M ± SD).

Amplitude analysis allowed us to note a significant decrease in the strength of the N75-N100 wave response to the black-and-white stimulus in all clinical groups, averaging 3.3 μV with control values of 8.5 μV. **Figure 2** shows a graphical representation of the VEP components.

Of greatest research interest was the analysis of the results obtained for the colour-changing checkerboard pattern. In the second trial, a reversal of red and yellow colours with a close range of visible light (red – wavelength 625-740 nm, yellow – wavelength 565-590 nm) was used. The conducted studies revealed reliable changes in both LP indices and response amplitude. The red-yellow reversed checkerboard pattern is presented in **Figure 3**.

The results of the study for the red-yellow reversed checkerboard pattern in terms of latent period and amplitude are presented in **Table 3**.

We noted that the most marked deviations in VEP parameters were reliably ($p < 0.01$) observed in patients with SPMS. Thus, the LP of the N75 wave was 91,850,53 ms, the LP in RMS and PPMS was significantly ($p < 0,01$) higher and

	N	Размах	Minimum	Maximum	Sum	Mean		SD	Dispersion	Asymmetry		Excess	
	Statistic	Statistic	Statistic	Statistic	Statistic	Statistic	SE	Statistic	Statistic	Statistic	SE	Statistic	SE
RMS	31	14	82	96	2776	89,55	,499	2779	7723	-,225	,421	1155	,821
SPMS	13	7	89	96	1194	91,85	,529	1908	3641	,598	,616	,480	1191
PPMS	16	4,00	86,00	90,00	1415,0	88,4375	,302	120,934	1463	-,738	,564	-,672	1091
N of valid(entirely)	13				0		33						

Table 2.
Results of descriptive statistics for VEP indicators for the black-and-white reversal pattern (wave N 75).

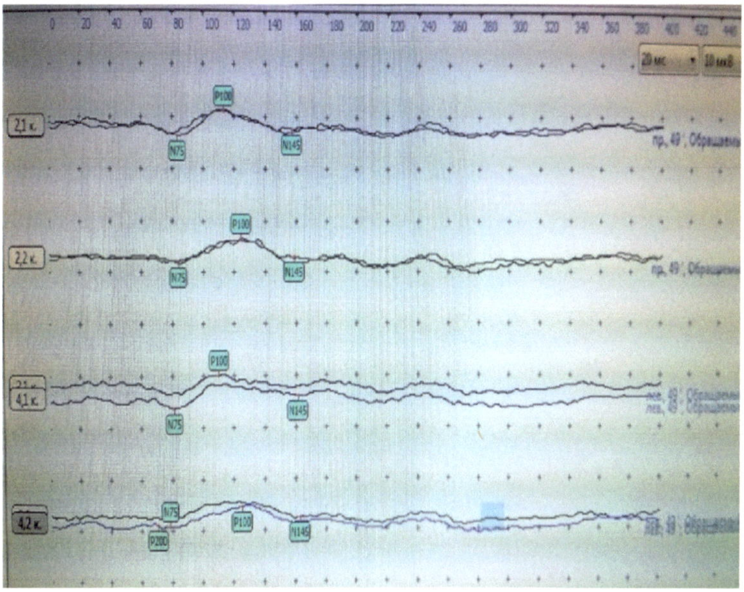

Figure 2.
Components of VEP on a reversed black-and-white checkerboard pattern. A 27-year-old patient with clinical form of SPMS.

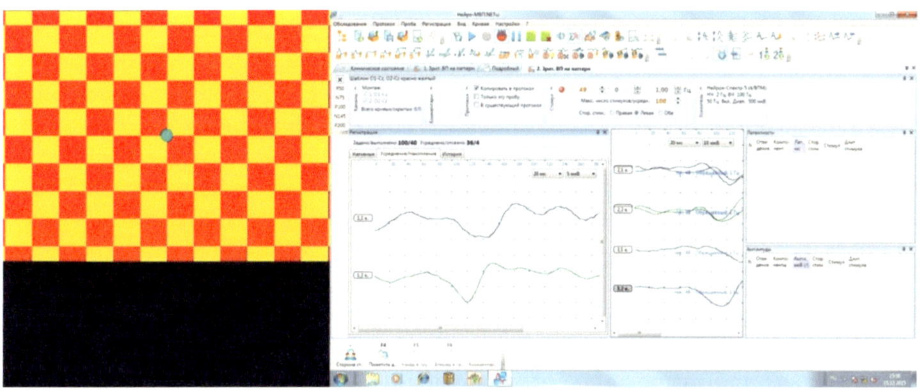

Figure 3.
Red-yellow reversed chess pattern.

was 89,550,49 ms in the first case and 88,840,25 ms in the second case (control group – 72,10,2 ms). The LP of the P100 wave was also sharply increased and significantly ($p < 0.001$) different from the control group, being 147.291.19 ms at RMS, 150.231.49 ms at SPMS, and 144.382.11 ms at PPRS (control group – 106.11.89 ms). The LP of wave N 145 was significantly higher than the control values. Correlation analysis (by Spearman) allowed us to note a significant correlation of the P100 wave predominantly with RMS and SPMS.

Amplitude analysis allowed us to note a significant decrease in the strength of the response to the red-yellow stimulus in all clinical groups, averaging 2 μV with control values of 8.5 μV.

According to the results on the green-black reversed checkerboard pattern, where the pulse exposure was directed in mono-colour mode of visible light and only

VEP indices	RMS n = 31	SPMS n = 13	PPMS n = 16	Control group n = 30
Latency period (ms)	89,55 ± 0,49	91,85 ± 0,53	88,84 ± 0,25	72,1 ± 0,2
N75	[88,53-90,57]*	[90,69-93,00]*	[88,30-89,38]*	106,1 ± 1,89
P100	147,29 ± 1,19	150,23 ± 1,49	144,38 ± 2,11	148,3 ± 1,41
N145	[144,86-149,71]*	[146,95-153,49]*	[139,78-148,98]*	8,5 ± 0,12
Amplitude (μV)	180,77 ± 0,98	180,30 ± 1,45	180,92 ± 1,70	
	[178,80-188,77]*	[177,14-183,47]*	[177,21-184,62]*	
	2,02 ± 0,07	2,00 ± 0,1	2,12 ± 0,12	
	[1,88-2,16]*	[1,77-2,22]*	[1,85-2,38]*	
Spearman's correlation	c SPMS +1000**	c PPMS- 0,468	c RMS – 0,468	c RMS +0,170
P100 wave	c PPMS- 0,468	c RMS + 1000**	c SPMS – 0,468	c SPMS +0,170
	with control group	with control group	with control group	c PPMS +0,496
	+0,170	+0,170	+0,496	

*95% confidence interval for the mean value.
**significant correlation at the 0.01 level (one-sided).

Table 3.
Quantitative measures of VEP in patients with different clinical forms of MS per coloured (red/yellow) checkerboard pattern (M ± SD).

influenced the cone cell system with a wavelength range of 500-565 nm, which is shorter than the wavelength of red and yellow colours in this VEP green test, a significant ($p < 0.001$) increase in PL was found in all clinical forms of MS (**Table 4**). The most significant lengthening of the LP of the N75 wave was in SPMS- 93,850,50 ms. The results of LP in RMS and PPMS were similar, being 90.550.5 ms in the first case and 89.430.30 ms in the second, and significantly ($p < 0.001$) differed from those of the control group. The LP index of the P100 wave was increased significantly and differed markedly ($p < 0.001$) from that of the control group, being 148.381.21 ms in RRS, 152.241.51 ms in SPMS, and 145.561.73 ms in PPRS. (control group – 106,11,89 ms). The change in LP index of N 145 wave was also reliably changed. A meaningful correlation was found between the groups in terms of VEP between RMS and PPMS.

The use of the green-black reverse checkerboard pattern is illustrated in **Figure 4**.

Amplitude analysis allowed us to note a significant decrease in the amplitude of the N75-P100 wave on the green-black stimulus in all clinical groups, not exceeding 2 μV on average, indicating a state of weak reaction of the visual cortex. The analysis of correlation dependence in patients with different courses of MS on P100 parameters in relation to the control group is presented in **Table 5**.

The results of the study suggest that the decrease in the amplitude of the response according to the results of VEP in different colour wavebands is associated with a decrease in the impulse flow along the fibres of the visual analyser and, as a consequence, an increase in the latency period, leading to a decrease in the number of neurons that activate the cortical response to the stimulus. The increase of LP on the visual analyser in MS patients is a consequence of demyelination processes. In this regard, to clarify these mechanisms, we conducted immunological studies related to the clarification of the concentration of IgG antibodies to myelin basic protein (MBP) as a manifestation of chronic immunological reaction. At examination of 46 patients, it was revealed that the concentration of IgG antibody level to MBP significantly ($p < 0,001$) exceeded the level of the control group and was 782,9 ± 5,2 μg/ml (control group 50,1 ± 2,12 μg/ml). It should be noted that the increase of antibodies to MBP was detected in all cases.

VEP indices	RMS n = 31	SPMS n = 13	PPMS n = 16	Control group n = 30
Latency period (ms)	90,55 ± 0,5	93,85 ± 0,50	89,43 ± 0,30	72,1 ± 0,2
N75	[89,53-91,59]*	[92,69-95,12]*	[88,79-90,08]*	106,1 ± 1,89
P100	148,38 ± 1,21	152,24 ± 1,51	145,56 ± 1,73	148,3 ± 1,41
N145	[145,90-150,86]*	[148,96-155,48]*	[141,86-149,25]*	8,5 ± 0,12
Amplitude (μV)	181,78 ± 0,97	182,32 ± 1,49	181,87 ± 1,40	
	[179,77-183,67]*	[179,19-185,52]*	[178,87-184,87]*	
	1,82 ± 0,08	1,76 ± 0,06	1,95 ± 0,1	
	[1,68-1,96]*	[1,63-1,90]*	[1,73-2,17]*	
Spearman's correlation	c SPMS +0,996**	c PPMS -0,468	c RMS – 0,411	c RMS ++0,127
P100 wave	c PPMS – 0,411	c RMS +0,996**	c SPMS -0,468	c SPMS +0,288
	contr. Group	contr. Group	contr. Group	c PPMS ++0,030
	+0,127	+0,288	+0,030	

95% confidence interval for the mean value.
****significant correlation at the 0.01 level (one-sided).*

Table 4.
Dynamics of quantitative indices of VEP in patients with MS on coloured (green/black) checkerboard pattern (M ± SD).

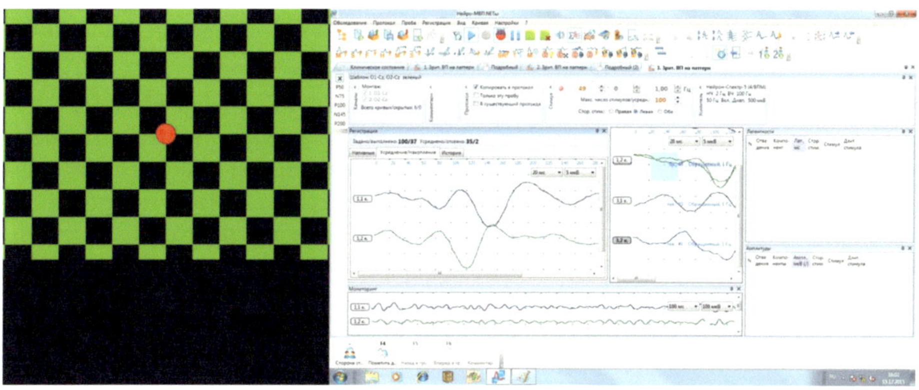

Figure 4.
Green-black reverse checkerboard pattern.

Thus, the results of the neurophysiological study demonstrate that in MS the processes of demyelination in the structures of the visual analyser are not identical for different light spectra. The most significant decrease in LP occurs on the colour spectrum of visible light relative to black and white, which can serve as an early diagnostic criterion in this disease. These changes lead to a sharp decrease in cortical response due to reduced axonal conduction along the fibres of the visual analyser. We believe that the use of the study results in clinical practice will greatly contribute to the improvement of early diagnosis of MS.

2.2 Analysing cognitive impairment using cognitive event-related potentials (P300)

We evaluated complaints about decreased concentration of attention and decreased memory, including long-term memory, which allowed us to identify the

		RMS 100	SPMS 100	PPMS P100	control
RMS P100	Pearson's correlation	1	,999***	-,435*	,204
	Significance(S).(one-sided)		,000	,046	,139
	N	31	13	16	30
SPMS P100	Pearson's correlation	,999**	1	-,444	-,270
	S.(one-sided)	,000		,064	,186
	N	13	13	13	13
PPMS P100	Pearson's correlation	-,435*	-,444	1	-,128
	S.(one-sided)	,046	,064		,318
	N	16	13	16	16
control	Pearson's correlation	,204	,270	-,128	1
	S.(one-sided)	,139	,186	,318	
	N	30	13	16	30

The correlation is significant at the 0.05 level (one-sided).
**The correlation is significant at the 0.01 level (one-sided).*

Table 5.
Correlation analysis in patients with different courses of MS according to P100 indices in relation to the control group.

degree of progression of disorders in the cognitive sphere in patients with MS. The analysis of endogenous P300 wave indices allowed us to objectively specify the degree of these disorders. The latency period is thought to be the time required to evaluate information, and the P300 amplitude is thought to reflect the relative amount of neural resources involved in processing the stimulus [4, 5]. Taking this into account, we found an increase in LP in all cases of patients with MS. The average LP results in different groups are presented in **Table 6**.

Thus, in the RMS group, the significant (p0.01) increase in the P300 wave was 323.13.11 ms in the SPMS group (p0.05) -345.13.11 ms, and in the PPMS group (p0.01) -337.52.45 ms. In a number of cases in both groups, we registered a slight increase in LP P300 with a decrease in the amplitude of the response, indicating an ambiguous course of neurophysiological changes in MS. It was noted that prolongation of LP P300 was noted predominantly in patients with SPMS.

The changed LP indices were reliably comparable in all studied groups. Perhaps this fact can be explained by the fact that different brain structures are involved in the formation of the cognitive wave, and in this regard, demyelinating processes in MS switch off certain areas and regions of neurons from the process of processing perception and analysis of information, thereby changing the formation of the positive P300 wave.

The results of P300 amplitude changes in both groups suggest that 'neuronal resources' are significantly involved in the pathological process in MS, with a tendency to decrease cortical activity as the pathology progresses. Thus, in the RRS group, the response amplitude was reduced and was 3.41.22 μV. In the RRS group, the amplitude was 2.91.52 μV, and in the PPRS group – 3.91.48 μV (control 5.20.61 μV). A positive correlation dependence of LP increase on MS disease duration was found.

The performed statistical analysis allowed to reveal a 2-sided correlation dependence at the level of 0.05 for LP, while no such dependence was revealed for the amplitude indices. This is graphically presented in **Figures 5** and **6**.

Age (years old)	RMS (n = 15)	SPMS (n = 11)	PPMS (n = 13)	Control (n = 31)
Latent period P300 ms	323,6 ± 3,79 ms [321,49–325,70]	345,1 ± 3,66 ms [342,54- 347,45]	337,7 ± 4,08 ms [335,18–340,12]	309,16 ± 1,37 ms [308,59-309,72]
Pearson's correlation S.(2-sided)	SPMS -,138 PPMS -,190 Control,129 SPMS,686* PPMS,535* Control,648*	RMS -,138 PPMS -,206 Control,284 RMS,686* PPMS,544* Control,397	RMS -,190 SPMS -,206 Control -,296 RMS,535* SPMS,544* Control,326	RMS,129 SPMS,284 PPMS -,296 RMS,648* SPMS,397 PPMS,326
Amplitude P300 (μV)	3,4 ± 0,25мкВ [3,21–3,48]	2,92 ± 0,25мкВ [2,70–3,03]	3,75 ± 0,36мкВ [3,48–3,92]	5,2 ± 0,09мкВ [5,12–5,19]
Pearson's correlation S.(2-sided)	SPMS -,074 PPMS,154 Control -,374 SPMS,829 PPMS,615 Control,170	RMS -,074 PPMS -,402 Control -,097 RMS,829 PPMS,220 Control,777	RMS,154 SPMS -,402 Control,579* RMS,615 SPMS,220 Control,038	RMS -,374 SPMS -,097 PPMS,579* RMS,170 SPMS,777 PPMS,038

*The correlation is significant at the 0.05 level (2-sided.)

Table 6.
P300 neurophysiological study indices depending on the course of multiple sclerosis.

Statistical analysis on the results of cognitive event-related potentials P300 points to the fact that there was a direct positive correlation (r = 0,36), where cognitive impairment according to P300 indicators depended mainly on the duration of the disease, which corresponded to the variants of MS course. Thus, the indices of latent period of P300 in SPMS were 346,433,62 ms (mean duration of disease – 9,1 ± 4,2 years), in RMS 335,473,69 ms (mean duration of disease – 3,3 ± 2,2 years), and in PPMS 332,483,88 ms (mean duration of disease – 2,7 ± 1,9 years) (control group – 309,161,37 ms).

To clarify the degree of cognitive impairment from among the most significant indicators of the cognitive wave P300 (ICW) we conducted a test of memorisation and reproduction of words. The studies of 39 patients using psychodiagnostic testing (PDT) allowed us to clarify the degree of processes of memorisation/remembering and reproduction of 10 words out of six attempts. Thus, in 4 (10.3%) cases the level of

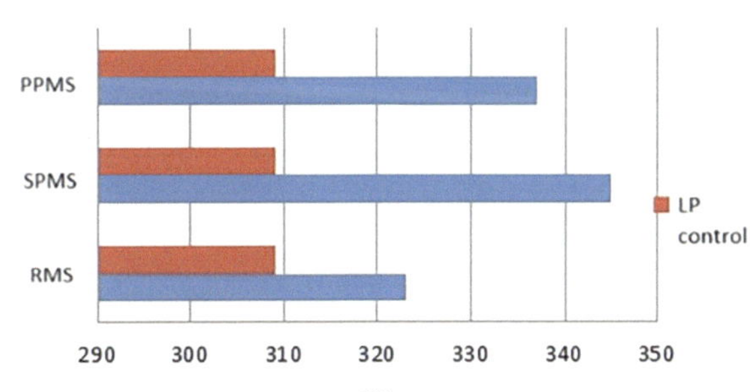

Figure 5.
Indices of latent period (LP) of P300 in patients with different course of MS in comparison with the control group (in ms.).

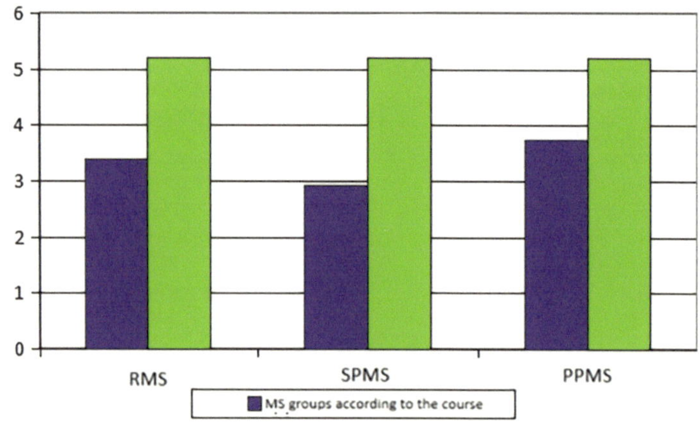

Figure 6.
P300 amplitude indices in patients with different course of MS in comparison with the control group (μV.).

memorisation was estimated as high (8 – 9 points), in 14 (35.9%) cases – average (6–7 points) and in 21 (53.8%) cases the level of memorisation processes was estimated as low (2–3 points).

Registration of cognitive event-related potentials of the brain to an auditory stimulus (P300) in these subjects made it possible to quantify the relative amount of neuronal resources involved in processing the stimulus. In the study, changes in amplitude and LP P300 indicated the interest of CNS structures responsible for the mechanism of information processing, where LP P300 values in patients with a score of 2-3 points were significantly (p0.01) increased and totalled 345.13.83 ms. In the group of patients with 6-7 scores PDT was also significantly (p0.05) increased and was 334.13.74 ms. In those cases when the PDT was a high score, the LP of the endogenous P300 wave was increased, but no reliable values were obtained. It should be noted that the amplitude index was slightly higher and was 4.11.24 μV than that of the control group. In this regard, when we talk about consciousness in the context of psychodiagnostics, we should mean arbitrariness, volitional internal control and speech-mediated basic conscious processes, such as perception, memory, attention, imagination, and thinking. The analysis of comparison of neurophysiological results on the P300 cognitive wave with PDT indicators allowed us to compare objective and subjective indicators of cognitive functions of the brain in MS and to confirm the fact that in the demyelinating process, there is a disruption of analytical functions of the CNS. Correlation analysis revealed a positive correlation between the dependence of a low PDT score and an increase in LP ($+0.52 \pm 0.13$). The revealed regularity indicates the dependence of the severity of learning/cognitive processes on the degree of axonal disorders, indicating the processes of demyelination in the CNS structures.

In addition, the presence of cognitive impairments (CI) in MS was detected by the Clock-Drawing Test, which is the most accessible, simple and quick test for assessing the results. We noted an increase in the incidence of impairment in patients, mainly in the group with SPMS and PPMS, with statistically reliable $p < 0.05$ results for this test.

Central myelin basic protein (cMBP) is a highly immunogenic protein, and autoimmune reactions are targeted at it during immune aggression. Immunological examination was carried out to detect the concentration of IgG in the central basic protein of myelin. In 46 patients with MS the concentration of IgG to cMBP

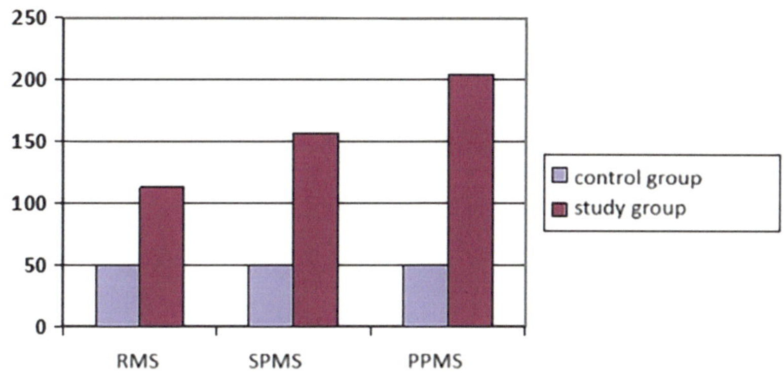

Figure 7.
The ratio of antibodies to cMBP in the studied groups and the control group.

significantly ($p < 0.05$) exceeded the level of the control group and was 112.6 ± 4.1 μg/ml in the RMS group, 156.5 ± 6.1 μg/ml in the SPMS group, and 204.4 ± 7.1 in the PPMS group (control group 50.1 ± 2.12 μg/ml), as shown in **Figure 7**.

It is noted that an increase in the titre of antibodies to cMBP was found in all cases. It should also be noted that a low titre of cMBP is a consequence of an inactive demyelinating process at the time of immunological examination. At the same time, single analyses taken from patients at the time of demyelinating process exacerbation indicated a high titre of cMBP, amounting in some cases to 650 μg/ml and more, which may require further investigation of immunological samples in different MS courses during demyelinating process exacerbation.

3. Results and discussion

The analysis of the data obtained in the present study showed a more pronounced improvement of the neurological status in patients who received, in addition to the standard treatment regimen, cytoflavin.

Thus, in the second group, the majority (89.5%) of patients normalisation of tendon reflexes, reduction of spasticity in the limbs and stabilisation of coordination disorders were noted. At the same time, in group 1 patients who received only basic therapy, positive neurological dynamics were revealed in 68,2% of patients and had a less pronounced picture – reduction of neurological deficit, mainly in the coordinator sphere ($p \leq 0,01$).

Positive dynamics of the visual analyser function were revealed in 63,2% of patients in group 2 and in 59,1% in group 1 ($p > 0,05$).

More frequent (1.7 times) absence of positive response to the treatment was revealed in group 1 patients in comparison with group 2 patients (18.2 vs. 10.5% respectively, $p \geq 0.03$). In the dynamics of observation, it was noted that the therapeutic effect of inclusion of cytoflavin in the therapy scheme started after 10 days of the drug administration and was sufficiently persistent – it persisted for more than 4 months after the end of the treatment course. There were no adverse events when taking cytoflavin, and all patients received treatment in full.

Thus, according to the results of the present study, we can conclude that the inclusion of cytoflavin as a drug with antioxidant and neuroprotective effect in the standard scheme of therapy for patients with MS in the exacerbation stage increases its effectiveness. This is manifested by more pronounced positive dynamics of neurological symptoms (reduction of pyramidal disorders – normalisation of tendon reflexes, weakening of spasticity in the limbs and stabilisation of coordination disorders), restoration of the function of the visual analyser and fewer cases of non-response to treatment. The results of the study confirm the previously obtained data; therefore, the prescription of cytoflavin is justified in terms of efficacy and safety and can be recommended for use in this category of patients.

4. Conclusion

Thus, the clinical and neurophysiological examination of MS patients revealed that patients with RMS were predominantly those whose clinical EDSS score corresponded to a mild degree of disability. Neurophysiological indices of evoked visual potentials on the colour pattern indicate that in MS in the structures of the visual annalisator the earliest disturbances occur on the short-wave spectrum of visible light, which may serve as an early diagnostic criterion in the diagnosis of the demyelinating process.

An objective study using cognitive evoked potentials (P300) indicates that cognitive impairment depends predominantly on the duration of the disease. A decrease in the amplitude of the P300 wave response indicates an insufficient number of neurons involved in signal processing and, therefore, a rearrangement of neuronal ensembles in MS, allowing us to quantify the state of neuronal relationships in signal processing and to clarify the nature and severity of neurophysiological shifts in the CNS in MS.

Acknowledgements

The authors are personally grateful to Petr Shevchenko, Evgeniya Nazarova, Irina Dolgova for their assistance in conducting this study and writing this article. The authors also express special gratitude to Milana Alibekovna Sultanbekova, a student of the Faculty of Medicine of Stavropol State Medical University, for productive co-operation, translation and editing of this article.

Conflict of interest

The authors declare no conflict of interest.

Author details

Sergey Mikhailovich Karpov* and Irina Andreevna Vyshlova
Department of Neurology, Neurosurgery and Medical Genetics, Stavropol State Medical University, Stavropol, Russia

*Address all correspondence to: karpov25@rambler.ru

References

[1] Karpov SM, Pazhigova ZB, Karpova EN. Visual evoked potentials in the study of the visual analyser in patients with multiple sclerosis. Neurology Neuropsychiatry Psychosomatics [Internet]. 2014;**3**:27-27. Available from: https://nnp.ima-press.net/nnp/article/view/433?locale=ru_RU

[2] Thompson AJ, Banwell BL, Barkhof F, Carroll WM, Coetzee T, Comey G, et al. Diagnosis of multiple sclerosis: 2017 revision of the McDonald criteria. The Lancet Neurology. 2018;**17**(2):162-173

[3] Nikolaevich BG. Multiple sclerosis: Diagnosis and pathogenetic therapy [Internet]. dissertat. 2024. Available from: https://www.dissercat.com/content/rasseyananny-skleroz-diagnostika-i-patogeneticheskу-terapiya

[4] Kutas M, McCarthy G, Donchin E. Extending mental chronometry: The P300 as a measure of stimulus evaluation time. Science. 1977;**197**(4305):792-795

[5] Isreal JB, Chesney GL, Wickens CD, Donchin E. P300 and tracking difficulty: Evidence for multiple resources in dual-task performance. Psychophysiology. 1980;**17**(3):259-273